PRAISE FROM PATIENTS FOR DF

"I suffered with back pain for nine years . . . [but now] I am working and living with the confidence that I can make it. There are so many people out there suffering in pain to the point of wanting to give up and die, like I felt. I want them to know how this procedure has changed my life."   —Daniel O.

"I was unable to perform many simple activities. The pain was a constant, always present companion in whatever I was doing . . . [but now] life is once again bliss. . . . Dr. Marcus is truly my hero."   —David W.

"Dr. Norman Marcus truly changed the quality of my life."   —Twinker M.

"I lived with extreme upper and lower back pain for three years. I was finally introduced to Dr. Marcus and after two weeks of treatment I am pain free."   —Clifford C.

"Dr. Marcus pinpointed the problem and treated it. He does not teach how to live with pain, instead he eliminates the pain."   —Yayoi S.

"Thanks to Dr. Marcus I have a much brighter outlook and look forward to more improvements to come."   —Alan O.

"To say that Dr   my l   inderstatement— they saved my '   —Christopher H.

"There is no b   r the   h   to back pain . . . after eleven m   ..   pain, tv   nt physical therapists, three co   e shots   laying basketball again within c   ..o   —Frank R.

PRAISE FROM DOCTORS FOR DR. NORMAN MARCUS AND *END BACK PAIN FOREVER*

"Professor Marcus came to England eighteen years ago and set the medical world alight with his clear thinking and non-operative approach to back pain . . . [this is an] excellent and highly readable book."

—Alan Bailey, MB, FRCP,
past chief medical advisor to Standard Life Healthcare

"Although designed for patients, many providers may find the text informative and change their current practices. This volume could be life saving for many patients with persistent back pain."

—Bill McCarberg, MD, founder of the Chronic Pain
Management Program, Kaiser Permanente, San Diego, CA

"Your back pain can be cured. Read this book. Dr. Norman Marcus eliminates low back pain by focusing on the major problem—muscle pain. His treatment and prescribed exercises work—I know because he treated and cured me."

—Thomas J.J. Blanck, MD, PhD; Dorothy Reaves Spatz,
MD Professor of Anesthesiology, Physiology, and Neuroscience;
chairman, Department of Anesthesiology, NYU Langone Medical Center

"Impressive and unusual in many ways: it is comprehensive, tries to present even basic data in a way that can be understood by the laymen, and offers not only [his] treatment method but also exercises for the patient. All in all: well done!"

—Siegfried Mense, MD, University of Heidelberg,
medical faculty at Mannheim, Neuroanatomy

"The treatment of back pain in America has suffered from weaknesses of diagnosis and a poverty of effective treatments. This volume . . . brings intelligence and clarity to an area that profoundly needs such an activity."

—Robert Cancro, MD, Lucius N. Littauer
Professor of Psychiatry and chairman emeritus

Also by Norman Marcus, MD

Freedom from Pain

End Back Pain
FOREVER

A Groundbreaking Approach to Eliminate Your Suffering

Norman Marcus, MD

ATRIA PAPERBACK

New York   London   Toronto   Sydney   New Delhi

To Hans Kraus, Siegfried Mense, and Suzy

ATRIA PAPERBACK
A Division of Simon & Schuster, Inc.
1230 Avenue of the Americas
New York, NY 10020

First Atria Paperback edition June 2012

ATRIA PAPERBACK and colophon are trademarks of Simon & Schuster, Inc.

For information about special discounts for bulk purchases, please contact Simon &
Schuster Special Sales at 1-866-506-1949 or business@simonandschuster.com.

The Simon & Schuster Speakers Bureau can bring authors to your live event. For
more information or to book an event, contact the Simon & Schuster Speakers
Bureau at 1-866-248-3049 or visit our website at www.simonspeakers.com.

Designed by Timothy Shaner, nightanddaydesign.biz

Manufactured in the United States of America

10   9   8   7   6   5   4   3   2   1

Library of Congress Cataloging-in-Publication Data
Marcus, Norman J.
  End back pain forever: a groundbreaking approach to eliminate your suffering /
Norman J. Marcus.
     p. cm.
1. Backache—Treatment. 2. Backache—Physical therapy. 3. Backache—Exercise
therapy. I. Title.
  RD768.M383 2012
  617.5'64062—dc23

                              2012007038

ISBN 978-1-4391-6744-1
ISBN 978-1-4391-6745-8 (ebook)

The information and advice presented in this book are not meant to substitute for the advice of your physician or
other trained healthcare professionals. You are advised to consult with healthcare professionals with regard to
all matters that may require medical attention or diagnosis and to check with a physician before administering or
undertaking any course of treatment.

Contents

CHAPTER 1

"Doctor, My Back Is Killing Me!"

You feel a twitch in your low back, then a heaviness and a sudden stab of pain. It strikes without warning: when you are crossing the street, stacking the dishwasher, jogging, whacking a golf ball, lifting a baby, swatting a fly, carrying groceries, bending over, getting out of a car, or just turning on a faucet.

Now you're afraid to move. You're locked in place. You feel a belt of pain pulsing across your back from hip to hip. You wonder, "What's happening? What did I do to get this?" You feel as though you're cut in half, as the pain seems to separate you from your legs. "Will the pain go away? Will it stay?" Gingerly, you start to move, but the pain only strikes harder. No, it's not going away, not at all. And if—this is a big "if"—the pain does ease off in a few days or go away in a couple of weeks, studies show that over time, it is certain to return in close to 50 percent of patients.

Back pain can be your personal bully. It can readily become chronic, lasting for months, years, even a lifetime. It may become so intense and disabling that your life can change dramatically for the worse. It can strip you bare financially, isolate you from family and friends, and leave you anxious and depressed. It can banish even the mere thought of sex. The curious thing about pain is that the more you think about it, the worse it becomes. Preoccupied with your pain, you lose interest in hobbies and sports. Your decreased activity may lead to obesity, which, in turn, can increase your chances of developing diabetes and heart disease. You watch in despair as you decline physically, mentally, and spiritually.

This book means exactly what the title *End Back Pain Forever* says. I have written it so that you can end your back pain once and for all and avoid a life of despair. I say this as a physician who has treated more than ten thousand patients in thirty-five years of private practice and as a past president of the American Academy of Pain Medicine, the medical society that represents physicians practicing a multidisciplinary approach to the treatment of pain.

I have seen many patients so wracked by pain that they wished they were dead, and some who actually attempted suicide before they saw me. So I am aware of the helplessness that you and millions like you feel when you first hobble into the doctor's office and exclaim, "Doctor, my back is killing me! I can't go on like this!"

Let me describe a common scenario: after some pokes and prods, the doctor says, "Go home, take an aspirin, lie down, and rest."

You do as the doctor says. But it does no good, and two days later, having missed work, you see the doctor again. "Well," says the doctor, "you have a case of nonspecific low back pain. We see a great deal of it."

The diagnosis sounds scientific, but it leaves you completely baffled and still wracked with pain.

"What does 'nonspecific low back pain' mean, Doctor?"

"It means that we don't know the cause."

"You don't know the cause?"

Should you ask more, you'll learn that nonspecific low back pain, also known by the acronym NSLBP, is so baffling that the International Association for the Study of Pain devoted an entire chapter to it in *Functional Pain Syndromes: Presentation and Pathophysiology*, a book for professionals published in 2009. The authors draw the frustrating conclusion that "it is exceedingly difficult to identify specific pathology underlying NSLBP." Of course, this is of no help to you or to anyone else.

"I can put you on strong medication to dull the pain," says the doctor. "It may be that your spine is the problem."

"Does that mean surgery?"

"It could. Surgeons do a million spinal operations a year."

Surgery on your spine is the last thing you want to do, but your back pain is horrendous. And, of course, you want to get better. So you say, "Can't we do an MRI or a CT scan to see if there's anything wrong with my spine?" MRI, or Magnetic Resonance Imaging, is a picture generated by magnetic fields, while a CT (computed tomography) scan is a picture generated by X-rays.

When you are shown the test results, the doctor points out that the images of your spine show that you have, say, a herniated disc (in which the cushion between two bony vertebrae is either protruding or has ruptured) or spinal stenosis (a narrowing of the spinal column that houses your spinal cord), or some other spinal anomaly—and that, apparently, is the cause of your pain.

But if it were true that the abnormality on the MRI or CT scan was indeed the cause of your pain, I wouldn't have written this book—because almost no one has a "normal" MRI or CT scan of the lower spine, and what is read as abnormal is frequently *not* the cause of your pain.

That bears repeating: when an MRI shows a herniated disc, it does not necessarily mean that the disc is causing your pain. Many people have a herniated or degenerated disc as a consequence of aging, and yet they have no back pain. Furthermore, it certainly does not mean that surgery is needed.

Actually, studies have shown that patients who get imaging tests increase their chance of undergoing an invasive treatment such as surgery or spinal nerve injections. Studies have also shown that when an MRI or CT scan for back pain indicates that something is "wrong" with the spine, patients are left to believe they will never truly be "normal" again, regardless of whether their pain is ever reduced or eliminated through any form of treatment. And bear in mind that as many as half of all spinal operations fail.

In fact, *the primary source of 75 percent or more of all back pain is from the muscles, not the spine.* In 2001 a study of more than twenty thousand patients at outpatient medical clinics in the United States found that sprains and strains of muscles and other soft tissue accounted for 70 percent to 80 percent of all back pain. This is strikingly similar to the findings of a study of three thousand patients with back pain conducted at Columbia Presbyterian Medical Center in New York City in 1946, which revealed that weak and stiff muscles were the source of pain in 83 percent of the participants.

It is truly astonishing that so many physicians who treat back pain have failed to make use of these findings. For years, medical schools have paid very little attention to the muscular system, even though muscles account for approximately half the weight of the body. Medical practice in recent decades has relied increasingly on high-tech imagery for diagnosis. Although high-tech imagery is certainly of great value—as is surgery, when required—neither X-rays nor MRIs nor CT scans are designed to detect the subtle nuances associated with muscle as a source of pain.

Take the case of a patient whom I shall call Stephanie. She is a married attorney who in 2004 began to experience stiffness whenever she got up out of a chair. She also had problems straightening up if she bent over. This was bothersome, but it was nothing compared to her first attack of spasms in her low back, on the right side. The spasms were incapacitating. She couldn't walk and had to lie in bed for four days, taking painkillers and muscle relaxants. When the spasms broke, she still felt an inkling of discomfort that would frequently and unexpectedly morph into repeat episodes of painful spasms.

It was during one of these crippling occasions that Stephanie went to a major teaching hospital, where an orthopedic surgeon ordered an MRI. The results showed that a disc in her lower spine was flattened, and the surgeon felt that the best treatment for this condition, called *degenerative disc disease* (DDD), would be a lumbar disc replacement. Stephanie wanted a less aggressive treatment and saw another surgeon, who referred her to a *physiatrist* (a doctor who treats physical impairments and disabilities). The physiatrist felt that her problem arose from one of the small joints in her spine, known as *facet joints*, rather than from the DDD. He treated her with injections of a local anesthetic to block the nerve that innervates the facet joint, which relieved some of her pain. Since the *nerve block* had proved partly successful, Stephanie's doctor suggested that the nerve be "turned off" temporarily with a procedure known as *radiofrequency ablation.* The physician would make a small incision in the skin and then use a handheld probe to deliver radio waves to the offending nerve, heating it until it can no longer transmit pain signals. Fearful of tampering with her nerves, Stephanie rejected this option. With no other conventional pain treatment options, and although there was no good indication for it, she agreed to an epidural steroid injection into her lower spine but this was ineffective. Five courses of *physical therapy* were also unsuccessful, and some of the sessions made her feel worse.

Stephanie first saw me in 2006 during one of her periods of muscle spasms. Her pain was so severe that she had been unable to work for two weeks. The pain had spread on this occasion from her right low back to both sides of her back and buttocks, with pain going to her hips and groin and also to her lower legs, feet, and toes. It consisted of a dull ache in her legs and a sense of pressure in the region of her spine. Her family, alarmed by the severity of the attack, urged her to finally have back surgery and "get it over with once and for all." Since she needed to "fix" the "damaged" disc sometime, why not now?

I examined her with an electrical instrument I devised that can identify specific muscles causing pain. This device works by stimulating a specific muscle to contract. If that contraction produces pain, it suggests that that muscle is a source of your pain. Using electrical stimulation, I determined that five muscles in her low back and buttocks were tender. But continued stimulation reduced the pain and actually eliminated it in most of the muscles. This told me that it was her muscles causing the pain, and that it was due to spasms, tension, and stiffness. I treated her with my spasm protocol: electrical stimulation to fatigue the muscle, followed by a different form of electrical stimulation to make the muscle move gently, followed, in turn, by gentle limbering exercises that I will teach you in Chapter 10.

After Stephanie's first visit, her pain was reduced by 60 percent. She returned for two additional sessions to relieve the spasm and was taught all twenty-one exercises found in Chapter 10. This brought her total relief. She now does the exercises every day, and four years later remains completely pain free.

Stephanie had "abnormal" findings on her MRI. Nerve blocks to the facet joints of her spine had managed to relieve some of her pain. But with my treatment, she never needed or had a disc replacement or long-term blocking of the nerves that serve her facet joints. She had received a host of well-meaning, costly interventions and suggestions for even more. But all of her pain could have been treated from the start simply, inexpensively, and safely by addressing tense, stiff muscles.

Given Stephanie's previous experience with doctors, she well understands the quotation that hangs on my office wall. It is from Eugene Bauer, an internist at the University of Vienna Medical School, who said in 1931, "A word in the mouth of a physician is as dangerous as a scalpel in the hands of a surgeon."

By showing her the results of X-rays and MRIs, her doctors led her to believe that she was permanently damaged goods. What they saw on the MRI was definitely there. But in her case, as in so many others, the true source of her pain was elsewhere: in her muscles. The truth is that without a muscle examination, we do not have an accurate explanation for your pain or anyone's pain.

My professor of anatomy at SUNY Upstate Medical University, Philip Armstrong, MD, used to say, "Reiteration without irritation is the essence of good education," and so to repeat the mantra for you: *the primary source of 75 percent or more of all back pain is from the muscles, not the spine.*

CHAPTER 2

You Are Not Alone:
The Back Pain Epidemic

If you suffer from back pain, you are not alone. The widespread failure by doctors to recognize muscles as the primary source of back pain is helping to fuel an epidemic. Back pain is now the most common disability in the United States. Every year twelve million Americans make new-patient visits to physicians for back pain and a reported one hundred million visits to chiropractors. At the current rate, eight out of ten Americans will experience back pain sometime during their lives.

In addition to the human suffering, medical costs are soaring. The cost of back pain, together with related neck pain, came to $86 billion in 2005, the most recent year for which figures were available. That was an increase of $34 billion from 1997. More amazingly, 25 percent of patients reported being significantly impaired, compared with 20 percent eight years earlier. Spending on back pain now equals the amount spent on cancer and is largely the result of failed surgeries, various nerve block procedures, and the cost of pain medications. We are spending more and getting worse results.

Back pain is not only a challenge to civilians, it is one of the major reasons for loss of combat personnel in the army. Disease and nonbattle injuries have always caused more casualties than battle-related injuries. Currently, low back pain is the most common disabling complaint among soldiers in combat, and it is more likely to result in a soldier never returning to active duty than any other diagnosis, except psychiatric. Recent studies have shown that of soldiers disabled by back pain, only 2 percent returned to duty with their unit.

Why have you and millions like you been caught in this epidemic? The reasons are both obvious and subtle. The luxuries of modern society, not only in the United States but also in all advanced countries, just about guarantee that you will suffer back pain because you are (1) under-exercised and (2) subjected to stress.

Muscles are strong and limber only when exercised properly. Lack of exercise makes them weak, short, and stiff, all of which help cause back pain, neck pain, and other muscle pain. The fact that 63 percent of Americans are overweight is one indication that the majority of the population does not exercise sufficiently. Another is the multitude of labor-saving devices and conveniences that reduce our physical activity—cars, snowblowers, lawn tractors, vacuum cleaners, dishwashers, to name a few—not to mention computers and television, which seduce us into inactivity.

About 30 percent of the population participate in exercise of some kind: tennis, swimming, jogging, lifting weights, and so on. This reduces the risk of developing back pain but is no guarantee against it. After all, professional athletes, from tennis stars to major league baseball players, are often afflicted with back pain. In their case, lack of exercise is not the issue, but rather improper stretching or insufficient warm-ups and cooldowns, in addition to injuries.

Compounding the problem is stress, which occurs in two forms: external and internal. External stress can come from the frustration you may feel sitting in a traffic jam or being subjected to an automated telephone menu. It may be brought on by irritating noises—a neighbor's loud music, jackhammers tearing up the street—or perhaps by your anger at rude service in the supermarket. Internal stress comes largely from anxiety. Ordinary worries about any number of concerns in daily life—jobs, rent, mortgage payments, grades, health, sex—can bring it on.

In 1915, Dr. Walter B. Cannon of Harvard Medical School, who made significant contributions to medicine, was the first to use the engineering term "stress" in an emotional context. He found that when an animal is threatened or irritated, it releases the hormone adrenaline (also known as epinephrine) into the bloodstream, causing a rise in respiration, heart rate, blood pressure, and blood sugar, and increases muscle tension. The animal then fights or flees, discharging the energy that came from its preparation to ward off the threat. When the challenge is over, its body returns to normal.

Although we humans are animals, we do not respond the way that other animals do. Society demands that we bear with our external and internal stress. We don't have the opportunity to fight or take flight to relieve our tension. As the stress builds day after day, it increases the tension on our already under-exercised, weak, short, stiff muscles. I will talk more about stress and its effect on pain in Chapter 7.

As a physician specializing in pain medicine, I know how intimately mind and muscles interact. I can literally see a patient's mental stress in tense, taut muscles. Early on in my training at Montefiore Medical Center in psychosomatic medicine, which is the study of how the mind and body interact, I could see that the separation of mind and body in medical practice made little sense. This drew me to a newly introduced technology, biofeedback, which enabled me to integrate my medical education with my psychiatric practice at the time.

The term "biofeedback" means measuring a function of the body—for example, temperature of the skin, heart rate, or muscle tension—and providing feedback in terms of sound, light, or a meter reading that reflects whether those physiological elements are increasing or decreasing. This is done by attaching a probe to your finger that senses temperature change, a probe to monitor heart rate, or an electrode attached to the muscle that you wish to study that senses electrical activity in that muscle—these electrodes lead into the device that gives you the feedback and makes you more aware of the changes occurring. With that information, you can actually raise the temperature of your skin, lower your heart rate, or lower muscle tension, all of which have been associated with producing relaxation and decreasing various pains.

Thus, if you are attached to a biofeedback device and asked, for example, about something you dislike, you may see your muscle tension and heart rate go up, while your skin temperature goes down. These changes suggest that you are experiencing stress or tension in your body, and that a part of your nervous system called the *sympathetic nervous system* is being stimulated. The sympathetic nervous system controls the heart and blood vessels and is generally stimulated when we are anxious or stressed. With practice, patients can be taught and eventually can teach themselves, by trial and error, how to control their physiological responses to emotions, thereby reducing the muscle tension that generates pain.

In 1975, I became a staff physician in the Montefiore Department of Neurology's Headache Unit, founded by Dr. Arnold Friedman. Two years later, with Dr. Edith Kepes, an anesthesiologist at the hospital, we started the first outpatient pain center in New York City, effectively following the lead of Dr. John J. Bonica, a medical giant to whom we owe the study of pain as a recognized discipline. As a young army anesthesiologist during World War II, he pioneered pain-relieving techniques and treated ten thousand wounded soldiers. Dr. Bonica went on to write a 1,500-page medical classic, *The Management of Pain.* Dr. Kepes and I began a team approach with practitioners from different fields—including colleagues from anesthesiology, neurology, orthopedic surgery, neurosurgery, physiatry, psychiatry, and psychology—all of whom were interested in what could be done for patients tormented by chronic pain.

I subsequently expanded on this concept by starting the New York Pain Treatment Program at Lenox Hill Hospital in 1983. It was considered a state-of-the-art treatment center in a hospital setting, with an integrated team that involved not only doctors but also physical and occupational therapists, psychologists, and pain rehabilitation nurses. We used a variety of treatments: biofeedback and *relaxation training*; physical therapy to increase strength, mobility, and endurance; hypnosis to help control pain; stress management to provide coping skills for handling daily upsets that may increase muscle tension; *occupational therapy* to teach patients how to complete their routine tasks effectively through proper time management; individual, family, and group *psychotherapy* to resolve personal difficulties related to living with chronic pain; and medication management to eliminate many ineffective drugs that patients were taking in their journeys from doctor to doctor.

But our program had a basic flaw. We were convinced that teaching people how to live with their pain was usually the best we could do. We didn't believe that we could *eliminate* their pain. Many of our patients remained on strong medication indefinitely. If a patient had a 35 percent decrease in pain, I considered that good. If we got it down to 50 percent, it was considered a success.

Along with the vast majority of physicians, I was committed to the fallacy that most chronic pain couldn't be cured. Then, in 1993, I met Dr. Hans Kraus.

He was to transform my life and the lives of my patients. He was eighty-five years old and had just retired from his practice as a specialist in physical medicine and rehabilitation. He had also given up mountaineering and rock climbing. In all those pursuits, he had won international acclaim. Originally trained as an orthopedic surgeon at the University of Vienna, Dr. Kraus was well known for having successfully treated President John F. Kennedy's back pain after all prior treatments had failed. Yet his nonsurgical approach to treating patients with muscle pain, especially low back pain, was not accepted by other doctors, including some of the very doctors who referred their own patients to him for what proved to be successful treatment.

For example, one prominent orthopedic surgeon at the Columbia University School of Medicine, Dr. Frank Stinchfield, who routinely sent many of his back pain patients to Dr. Kraus, underwent spinal surgery rather than consult him for his own back pain after a herniated disk was diagnosed. The surgery failed, and Dr. Stinchfield was never able to work again because of unrelenting pain.

Another disappointing example was that of Dr. Jonas Salk, best known for developing the first safe and effective polio vaccine. Dr. Salk *did* consult Dr. Kraus for back pain, and the treatment *was* successful. It eliminated Dr. Salk's pain and allowed him to avoid surgery. Yet when Dr. Kraus needed Dr. Salk's help to obtain research support, the famed medical researcher declined. He said that muscle pain didn't have a "scientific foundation." That has since changed, and we will look at the basic research explaining the mechanisms of muscle pain in Chapter 4.

In our first meeting, Dr. Kraus asked what I did. I told him that I treated patients with chronic pain.

"How do you do that?" he asked.

"I teach them how to manage their pain, how to deal with it, live with it."

"Why not get rid of their pain?"

"Because it's chronic pain," I said. "You can sometimes reduce it, but you can't get rid of it."

He persisted. "Have you treated the muscles?"

"We treat the muscles with aerobic exercises."

"Aerobic exercises? Really? Muscle pain caused by muscle spasm, tension, stiffness, and trigger points does not respond to aerobics. But it will respond to other types of exercises: prescribed exercises designed to treat the specific source of pain. That's what I've done."

"Low-impact aerobics are the standard way," I said.

"They may be the standard way," he replied. "But they are sure to make many of your patients feel worse."

He asked if I had "very difficult cases," and I told him that I did. "Some," I added, "are impossible to treat."

"Would you mind if I were to examine one of them?"

Dr. Kraus and I met a week later at Lenox Hill. I had chosen a patient whom I shall call Beth. She was a forty-five-year-old woman so defeated by pain after three unsuccessful spinal operations that she could no longer hold a job. Her life had revolved around her work, which was at the core of her sense of self. She was devastated. No one had found a truly successful treatment for her, and I did not believe that anyone could. She was on high doses of morphine, 60 milligrams orally five to six times a day, to relieve her pain.

After reviewing her case history, Dr. Kraus gave her a comprehensive and thoughtful mental and physical examination. Starting with her neck, he used his fingertips to palpate her muscles to distinguish between those that were supple and pain free and those that were stiff and painful. He found five pairs of painful muscles on both sides of the lower back, buttocks, and thighs. "If these muscles are treated properly," he told me, "it should reduce or eliminate her pain."

I couldn't believe that this would be the case. Her diagnosis was arachnoiditis, inflammation of the deep layer of the membranous tissue surrounding the spinal cord. In Beth's case, it was caused by the dye that radiologists use to outline the spinal cord when performing a special X-ray called a myelogram. The oil-based dye used in the past sometimes irritated the tissue, producing scarring that could squeeze nerves and bring about pain in the back and legs. (Today a nonirritating water-based dye is used instead.) I knew that there was no good treatment, and Beth's future wasn't pretty. I had done my best to help her live with the pain in my pain management program. Even though she reported a 50 percent improvement, she was still taking large doses of morphine and couldn't return to work.

Beth and I had nothing to lose by trying. She demonstrated all of the reasons for muscle pain that I will explore with you as you get further into *End Back Pain Forever*. Beth was tense, weak, and stiff (deconditioned). She had areas of persistent painful contractions, or spasming, and tender spots in her muscles that Dr. Kraus knew from experience would respond to injections of lidocaine, a numbing solution. Beth would need prescribed exercises, but because her pain was so severe that all movement hurt, Dr. Kraus decided to start her treatment with injections into the identified painful muscles and then quickly add exercises.

The injection technique—different from the *trigger point injections* popular among other pain physicians—concentrated on the areas where the muscles attached to the tendon and the bone, in contrast to the tender nodules in the muscle tissue. (More on this later.) Only one muscle could be treated per day, and each injected muscle received three days of a special physical therapy protocol to restore its flexibility.

Four weeks later, the patient that I had considered "impossible to treat" returned to work free of pain. This was the most important medical awakening in my career.

Beth's arachnoiditis was a bona fide diagnosis. I had seen her CT scan following a myelogram. In fact, it had shown *severe* arachnoiditis. But her pain at that moment came from her muscles, not from her arachnoiditis. If we had not examined and found the painful muscles, she never could have been treated properly for the pain, and she would have been on the same medication, getting marginal results, for the rest of her life. It forced me to wonder how many other patients of mine were suffering needlessly because I had reflexively attributed their pain to their existing diagnoses, and whether they too were not receiving the proper treatment that could eliminate or diminish their suffering.

The successful resolution of Beth's case was such a revelation that I asked Dr. Kraus if he would be good enough to come to the Lenox Hill clinic for two hours once a week. He agreed, although that soon changed to one full day a week. He would come in at nine in the morning and leave at six. He did this for five years and quickly became a close friend and mentor.

I learned an extraordinary amount from Hans, all to the benefit of our patients, who began returning to normal lives following successful treatments that relieved their pain.

In 1993, the US Agency for Health Care Research and Policy convened a multidisciplinary medical panel to draw up guidelines for the treatment of low back pain. Hans and I went to Washington, D.C. and testified before the panel. One of the panel members, Dr. Richard Deyo of the University of Washington, had published a study that strongly indicated that one type of back surgery, *spinal fusion,* was often a poor choice. The panel suggested that surgery not be an option for most back pain in the first three months of an episode.

This prompted the surgeons in the North American Spine Society to accuse the panel of bias. The society had its way, and in 1995, despite objections by the American Medical Association, the American Hospital Association, and the American College of Physicians, Congress cut funding for the agency and eliminated the word "policy" from its name. In a compromise, a new agency took its place: the Agency for Healthcare Research and Quality, which was devoid of the power to suggest guidelines for treatment.

The number of back surgeries continues to rise. Today, in fact, back operations are by far the fastest-growing surgery in the country. There are now on the order of 400,000 back operations annually; 150,000 to 200,000 are spinal fusions. Additional studies have shown as many as half the operations are failures. A more measured, thoughtful approach than spine surgery could help patients suffering with back pain. But even many of the competing interventions, such as nerve blocks and nerve stimulation techniques, are bound to fail because they too are aimed at the wrong target.

The history of medicine is replete with examples of significant advances that were met with opposition, even ridicule, by the reigning authorities. Some were as sophisticated as the discovery of blood circulation, others as simple as the need for doctors to wash their hands. We can add to the list the fact that muscles, not spinal deformations, are the cause of most common back pain.

CHAPTER 3

Understanding Pain

This chapter describes the scientific mechanisms of how pain is produced and perceived. You may wish to reread this chapter later after learning more about back pain. If you want to dig in now, let me summarize what you will find. Pain may result from any damage to the body. Our understanding of the chemical reactions resulting from damage allows us to create drugs to block these effects. An example is aspirin. It blocks the formation of substances called prostaglandins, which are produced when a cell is damaged. Prostaglandins excite nerves that transmit signals that start a chain reaction of events that results in the brain being informed damage has occurred and may result in the experience of pain. This chapter gives an overview of that process.

The nature of pain has been a challenge to scientists and philosophers since at least the time of Aristotle. Since we experience pain in so many different ways, it has been called both a sensation and an emotion. Feeling the pain sensation is generally a reflection of some damage in your body. You cut your finger, and you report a sharp, burning pain. Some patients report their pain in language that is more extreme than the actual sensation caused by the damaged tissue. An example would be "This pain is killing me! It's torture!" You can probably guess that pain perceived as killing or torturing is harder to deal with than aching, burning pain and would result in you having a harder time functioning. Even though pain is generally the result of actual damage to a part of your body, you can also feel pain without any damage or injury; for example, when your heart "aches" because your best friend won't speak to you. The interaction of physical sensations with our general emotional state, which is affected by memories and current situations in our life, together form the experience we call pain. This topic is so important that Chapter 7 is devoted to the interplay of pain and emotions.

First let's try to understand how pain is a result of physical damage somewhere in the body.

Pain is a part of our life. It's an alarm signal that tells us something is wrong: "Stop! Get help!" It protects us from further harm. We need it as we grow up to learn about dangers in our surroundings. Congenital indifference to pain and congenital insensitivity to pain are two medical conditions in which a child is born with the inability to respond to injury. These children generally die by their teens due to the severe damage they inflict on themselves because they do not experience pain. Unlike them, should you fracture a bone in your ankle, the pain you would feel would stop you from putting weight on that ankle and causing further injury. We are programmed to recognize that pain means damage somewhere in our bodies. We call pain that has just begun *acute pain* and pain that continues for longer than expected *chronic pain*. Acute pain is the easier of the two to understand.

ACUTE PAIN

Whenever we damage anything in our body, we start a chain reaction that alerts our brain. Here is how it works: our bodies can be injured from a cut, bruise, tear, fracture, poison, lack of oxygen, and excessive heat or cold. Injured cells in the damaged tissue (bone, skin, muscles, tendons, ligaments) release chemicals. The body transforms some of these chemicals to substances that stimulate specialized nerves called *nociceptors,* which detect damage or the threat of damage (such as when you lift a heavy object and feel pain prior to actually damaging a muscle or tendon). There are many chemicals involved. Figure 1 in the insert depicts a very simplified version of what happens when a cell is damaged.

There are different types of nociceptors. They may respond to heat, mechanical stress, or increases in the amount of acid that occurs when tissue is damaged. The nociceptors send information to the spinal cord, which then sends the information to the brain. This allows you to recognize that an injury has occurred. The nerve that was stimulated by tissue damage releases a chemical called *Substance P* at the point in the spinal cord where the nerve attaches. Substance P stimulates other nerves in the spinal cord to continue transmitting information up to the brain, where we become conscious of the damaging event. See figure 2 in the photo insert for an illustration of this.

This information transmission process is simplified in figure 3 in the insert. The names of the pathways allow scientists to discuss and attempt to understand how and where the information is processed, and to find ways to reduce the pain.

Since this information is traveling from the body up to the brain, it is called *ascending,* or *afferent,* transmission. Fibers travel up into the lower parts of the brain (the *medulla* and the *pons*), then to the *midbrain,* and finally the *thalamus.* The major pathway going up toward the brain is called the *spinothalamic tract* because it connects the spine with the thalamus. The thalamus consists of a number of nerve bundles called nuclei, which interpret the information coming in and, much like a switchboard, direct the signals to other parts of the brain. Memories of past pain may be stored in the thalamus. Signals from the thalamus continue up to higher centers in the brain, including the *limbic system,* which is our emotional center, and the *sensory cortex,* where we localize the area that hurts. The limbic system compares this injury to others we have suffered, analyzes its impact on our life at the moment, and communicates back and forth with the sensory cortex, where we register where the injury occurred. When you have a pain that is similar to a past pain, the memory will help you manage the new pain, telling you, in effect, "It's only a slight bruise" or "Better get to an emergency room."

Impulses are also transmitted the other way: from the brain down to the body. This is called *descending,* or *efferent,* transmission. Descending transmission can exaggerate or minimize the flow of information telling us we have damage in the body. What this means is that the state of our brain (for example, being agitated and nervous or calm and peaceful) affects how we react to the damage and therefore how much pain we will experience. A calm doctor can create an air of confidence that is soothing, whereas an anxious caretaker can make your discomfort worse. Part of the process of increasing or decreasing your pain via the brain comes from the production of chemicals (endorphins, dynorphin, enkephalin, nociceptin/orphanin FQ) that are similar to the painkiller morphine. These can block the release of Substance P and decrease the sensations associated with tissue damage. Endorphins play a role in reducing pain and improving mood, but we still do not know their mechanism of action.

Some of the pain pills we take have actions similar to the body's painkillers. The strongest group of pain medications is called *opioids.* Common examples include Tylenol (acetaminophen) with codeine, Percocet (oxycodone and acetaminophen), Percodan (oxycodone and aspirin), and MSIR (morphine sulfate immediate release). These work by blocking the pain impulse in the spinal cord as well as stimulating an area in the midbrain called the periaqueductal gray to release a chemical called *serotonin*. This release results in the production of endorphin-like chemicals in the spinal cord, further blocking the pain signals where they first began. Cells called the locus coeruleus in the pons are sensitive to the chemical *norepinephrine,* while cells called the raphe nucleus in the medulla are sensitive to serotonin. Together these two chemicals, which are part of the family of nerve chemicals known as *neurotransmitters,* can suppress the pain signals. Since norepinephrine and serotonin are both involved, it suggests why drugs that increase only the available amounts of serotonin—*serotonin specific reuptake inhibitors* (SSRIs), such as fluoxetine (Prozac) and paroxetine (Paxil)—are not very effective for pain relief, whereas drugs that increase the availability of norepinephrine *and* serotonin—*serotonin-norepinephrine reuptake inhibitors* (SNRIs), such as amitriptyline (Elavil) and duloxetine (Cymbalta)—are effective. See figure 4 in the insert for more information.

The concepts of acute pain are complicated, and I present this simplified description only to show that we have some understanding of how pain is produced.

CHRONIC PAIN

When it comes to chronic pain, matters are even more complicated. The body generally heals from an injury in six weeks. If after that time you still have pain, where is it coming from?

Let's take an example that I can answer easily. Imagine having a broken bone in which the break went through a joint—let's say the hip joint. If the joint was damaged enough that it couldn't heal back to its normal shape, you might have persistent pain. Even if it did heal properly and cleanly, you could still at some point afterward have pain in the joint because breaks through a joint will often produce *arthritis,* an inflammation in the tissues that can be painful and limit motion. There is ongoing pain because the initial damage caused changes in your joint, which then became the new reason for ongoing pain.

But what about back pain? I will tell you in Chapter 6 how muscles are the reason for most acute and chronic back pain, but first let's look at how the medical community generally deals with back pain.

The majority of patients who complain of back pain are not found to have anything definitively wrong on their physical examination or imaging studies (X-ray, MRI, CT). I say "definitively wrong" because some professionals treating your back pain will claim that what they find on the physical and imaging examinations explains your pain, while others will say those same findings do not explain your pain. The majority of doctors will agree that when back pain begins, it is frequently impossible to find a simple reason for it. The pain may diminish, often striking again and frequently never going away entirely, all the while without any obvious cause. That's why it's called nonspecific low back pain. Your doctor's first job, when he sees you with back pain, is to make sure that the discomfort is not due to a serious condition. We call this investigation looking for red flags. If you can answer yes to all the questions below, you have no red flags, and you are considered at low risk for serious causes of back pain:

1. You're between ages eighteen and fifty.

2. Your pain is confined to the low back and buttocks and doesn't extend below the upper part of your thigh.

3. You have no consistent pain or loss of sensation in your legs.

4. Your pain is related to postural changes. For instance, it is worse when sitting, standing, or bending, so that some positions are better and others worse.

5. You are otherwise in good health.

If you answered yes to all the questions, no imaging studies are needed. Most often over-the-counter pain medications and possibly spasm-relieving drugs, along with being reasonably active, will be enough to help you manage until the pain disappears. But each negative question increases your chance of having more than just simple back pain that goes away by itself.

On the other hand, each item in the following history is a red flag—that is, it raises the suspicion that a specific cause of your pain might be found and should be treated:

1. Being over fifty gives you a greater chance of developing cancer or *osteoporosis* (weakened bones), and, therefore, a greater chance of having bone fractures. Cancer in your bones and fractures can both cause pain.

2. Having been involved in a serious accident such as a major fall on a hard surface or a car accident, which may have produced a fractured bone or torn ligaments and tendons.

3. A history of some disease such as diabetes or a previous bone infection (osteomyelitis), which could make you more likely to have an infection or bone-destroying condition. If you have cancer, your pain may be a sign

that it has spread to the area that hurts. Unexplained weight loss could be from undiagnosed cancer or infection.

4. Having an infection or a condition that is associated with a high chance of contracting an infection, such as AIDS, taking immunosuppressant drugs (for rheumatoid arthritis and other disorders), and intravenous drug abuse.

5. *Signs* (what we find when we examine you) and *symptoms* (what you report is troubling you) of nerve compression near your spine or pressure on the lower part of your spinal cord (the *cauda equina*), such as loss of sensation in your buttocks and your rectal and genital regions, along with problems controlling your bladder and rectum.

6. Pain that never lets up no matter how you position yourself.

7. Pain that continues to worsen over time.

Answering yes to any of these questions suggests that there is a chance of a serious underlying condition and that prompt additional testing is indicated. Fortunately, most patients with back pain are in the nonspecific, low-risk group.

We can look inside the body with X-rays, CT scans, and MRIs. Collectively, these tests are called imaging studies. You might be saying, "I have degenerative or bulging discs based on my imaging study, or another *specific* diagnosis, and that's why I have pain, so this doesn't apply to me." But, actually, it still does. As I have said, the diagnosis that you are given may be true in one sense. For example, an MRI may show a herniated disc—but it may not be causing your pain. An explanation of pain is frequently *not* a fact but an opinion. Two doctors may see the same evidence—diagnostic imaging, patient history, and physical examination—and come up with different diagnoses and treatment plans. Medicine is an art as much as a science. Doctors' conclusions concerning back pain are not based on guidelines derived from repeated successful studies of patients with back pain. Those studies don't exist. The studies that do exist and that are used to support some treatment for your back pain frequently show partial and/or temporary relief of pain, significant costs, and serious complications.

If you Google "back pain," you will come up with over sixty-nine million "hits." When you go to the various sites, you will find that many respected professionals (and nonprofessionals) have an explanation for why you might be suffering. The diagnosis you have been given is often based on an imaging study. I said before that these studies don't generally provide a reasonable *explanation* for your pain, but that doesn't mean they don't produce a *diagnosis*. In fact, they almost always provide some diagnosis such as spondylosis—which sounds ominous but means only that your spine doesn't look perfect. So many people have some imaging-based diagnosis without experiencing pain that it's not reasonable to assume that the same diagnosis is causing your specific pain. Here are some other common diagnoses:

- **Spinal, or foraminal, stenosis:** a narrowing of the openings in the bony spine that house the spinal cord and the nerves extending out from the spinal cord.

- **Facet arthropathy:** an overgrowth of bone and damaged cartilage of one of the joints that separates one spinal vertebra from another.

- **Spondylolisthesis:** slippage of one vertebra so that it does not sit evenly on the vertebra below it.

- **Degenerative disc disease:** a flattening of the disc-shaped tissue that separates and cushions two vertebrae.

- **Bulging or herniated disc:** when a spinal disc either protrudes abnormally or ruptures, leaking some of its gel-like contents.

If you assume that the cause of your pain can be explained based mostly on the diagnostic imaging without having considered muscles and emotional factors, you may miss the real cause of your pain, undergo the wrong treatment, risk additional damage, waste money and time, and needlessly perpetuate your pain and misery.

CHAPTER 4

Back Pain and Anatomy

Back pain is mentioned in medical literature as far back as 1500 BC in Egypt. Through the ages, various explanations have been offered for its cause and how to treat it. But it was not until the nineteenth century that the spine and the nervous system were seen as the fundamental source of back pain. The medical community adopted the idea that the cause of back pain was some injury to or irritation of the bones and nerves of the spine and this largely erroneous notion has persisted up to the present. Similarly, bed rest made sense to the majority of doctors, so it became a standard treatment through most of the twentieth century.

Some knowledgeable physicians recommended—even argued—that back patients should stay active. But their opinion was drowned out by proponents of bed rest, who insisted that back pain could take weeks to heal, and, therefore, patients should be hospitalized and often strapped in place to stretch the spine. This was a modern medical version of the medieval rack. Shackled patients were not allowed to get out of bed for a week or more. Only toward the end of the twentieth century did the medical community recognize that prolonged bed rest was damaging, by producing weakness and deconditioning, and that patients with typical back pain should be encouraged to remain active.

When X-rays were introduced around the turn of the twentieth century, doctors could see the joints in the spine and the pelvis, and they began to suggest that back pain originated from these parts of the body. New phrases such as "My sacroiliac is out" and "I have a bout of lumbago" crept into the language. A variety of spinal surgeries sprang up. The first report of spine surgery to remove a herniated disc to treat pain radiating down the leg (*sciatica*) came in 1934. In 1935 the same operation was suggested for back pain as well. Over the next twenty years, disc surgery became one of the most common operations performed by neurosurgeons.

ANATOMY OF THE SPINE

The spine consists of twenty-four interconnecting small bones in addition to the *sacrum*. These small bones are called vertebrae, and they are stacked on top of one another.

The spine has three sections: the *cervical spine* (neck), the *thoracic spine* (chest), and the *lumbosacral* spine (low back). The spine curves in the neck and low back, which is where the most wear and tear takes place and pain occurs most often. The vertebrae in the spine are numbered: cervical (C1–C7), thoracic (T1–T12), lumbar (L1–L5), and sacral (S1–S5, which are fused into one bone). See figures 5 and 6 in the color insert for visual representations of the spine.

PARTS OF THE BONY SPINE

The vertebrae are shaped so that they can both support the weight of the body and protect the spinal cord and spinal nerves. The part of the vertebra that bears most of the weight is called the *vertebral body*, which you can see by looking at figure 7 in the insert. Attached to the vertebral body and projecting backward are two plates of bone called the *pedicles*, which connect to another bony section, the *lamina*, together forming half an arch on either side. When the two lamina come together in the midline, an arch is formed (spinal canal), covering the spinal cord. Attached to the arch are two bony extensions that jut out from either side called the *transverse processes*.

The region where the lamina and the pedicle come together has specialized sections that allow the vertebrae above and below to form a joint. These sections are called the *inferior* and *superior processes*, and in a healthy spine, they are covered with cartilage and form four of the six joints found on each vertebra. There is a notch above and below each pedicle, which, when they come together in two adjacent vertebrae, forms a hole called the *intervertebral foramen*. Nerves that leave the spinal cord, called *spinal nerves*, pass through this foramen on their way out to various parts of the body.

THE JOINTS OF THE VERTEBRA

Two adjacent vertebrae will have three regions, called joints, where they touch each other. The largest joint is between the two vertebral bodies and actually has no formal name, but following the suggestion of Dr. Nikolai Bogduk, we will call them the *interbody joints*. The other two joints are formally called the *zygapophysial joints* and are more commonly referred to as the facet joints. Figure 8 in the insert shows two of the vertebral body's joints.

SPINAL DISCS

Sandwiched between each vertebra is a cushiony disc, which has at its center a jellylike substance with a high water content, called the *nucleus pulposus*. You can see it in figure 9 in the insert. The disc is covered by a very thick ligament known as the *annulus fibrosis* (see figure 10 in the insert), which connects the vertebral bodies of adjacent vertebrae. Two layers of cartilage on the top and bottom contain the disc and separate it from the vertebral body. Together the nucleus and the annulus act like a shock absorber and allow flexible movement of the spine.

SPINAL CORD AND NERVES

The nervous system functions to allow the recognition, collection, storage, and interpretation of information (facts, feelings, and memories), and to send and receive that information. It also transmits electrical impulses to and from different parts of the body to operate muscles and other organs. The nervous system is fragile and easily damaged. That is why the innermost parts of the nervous system, called the *central nervous system* (CNS), are covered by bone. The *brain*, which is the control center, is encased in the skull; the lower part of the CNS, the *spinal cord*, is encased in the bony spine. The vertebrae form a protective tunnel for the spinal cord, the thick bundle of nerves that is attached to the lower end of the brain, and ends in the lumbar spine. See figure 11 in the insert.

The nerves exit the spinal cord through the holes of the vertebrae, called foramen, and then travel to all parts of the body, allowing us to move our muscles, feel sensations, and automatically operate our bodily organs without conscious effort. Since the job of the nervous system is so complex, it is composed of different types of nerves to do different tasks. The organs of the body, such as the heart and the liver, need to work without any effort on our part. They are supplied by nerves that are part of the involuntary, or *autonomic, nervous system.* The nerves that allow us to be conscious of our surroundings, changes in our body, and movement are part of the *voluntary nervous system.*

NERVES CAUSING PAIN

If a nerve having a role in sensation is squeezed, it may produce an unpleasant sensation along its course. One way that pressure on the nerves and/or spinal cord can produce pain is when a herniated disc presses on a spinal nerve in your lumbar spine, causing pain to radiate down your leg. Figures 12 and 13 in the insert show this in detail.

More often, however, back pain will be the result of signals produced by damage to the soft tissue surrounding the spine. Muscles, tendons, and ligaments—the structures that are constantly moving and changing shape—are most often the generators of back pain. Stimulated pain fibers from these tissues transmit information to the spinal cord and up to the brain, where we feel the injury and associated pain.

CONNECTIVE TISSUE

Connective tissue is what joins parts of the body together. *Fibrous* connective tissue is one kind of connective tissue. There are three types of fibrous connective tissue: *ligaments, tendons,* and *fascia.* There are approximately thirteen ligaments that connect the vertebrae to each other and connect the lumbar spine to the hip bone (ilium). I say "approximately" because there is disagreement among anatomists as to what constitutes a ligament.

Muscles generally end in tendons, which then generally attach to a bone. Fascia encases all tissues of the body and sometimes connects muscle to muscle. If any fibrous connective tissue is damaged or about to be damaged by injury or overstretching, it can be a cause of pain.

LET'S TALK ABOUT MUSCLES

There are three types of muscles:

1. *Striated muscle*, also known as skeletal muscle, is under voluntary control and moves our body when we decide to perform a task. The word "striated" refers to the stripes that you see when you look at the muscle tissue under a microscope.

2. *Smooth muscle*, such as the muscle surrounding the intestines, is not under voluntary control.

3. *Cardiac (heart) muscle*, which is also striated, is not under voluntary control.

The muscles involved in back pain are striated. All further references to muscles in this book will be about striated muscle.

There are approximately 320 muscle pairs in the body, meaning the same muscle on the right and left side, and one unpaired muscle, for a total of approximately 641 muscles. I say "approximately" because some anatomists divide up muscles into different parts and give each a separate name, resulting in as many as 420 muscle pairs.

Muscles allow us to move. Complex movements (imagine LeBron James making a spinning jump and hook shot) are made possible because many muscles working together contract or relax in a pattern that produces the precise movement that we desire. Multiple muscles may work together even to perform what appears to be a simple movement.

When muscles are injured, they have an unusual quality. Pain may be experienced not only in the injured muscle, but it is also frequently *referred* to a muscle close by or even to a distant muscle. This mechanism of referred pain will be explained later in Chapter 5. Since almost any muscle can be a source of pain, it makes sense for both physicians and patients to learn as much as we can about each individual muscle in the region of the body where pain is felt. As an example, approximately eighteen muscles move the shoulder. Your doctor needs to know them all when trying to understand and treat upper and midback pain, and at least that many muscles for the low back and buttocks. A proper physical examination is the only way of determining which muscle in a painful region is a source of pain. A physician cannot find this out with imaging studies.

MUSCLES OF THE BACK

Let's look at what we would find if we peeled away the layers of the skin and connective tissue of the back down to the muscles to see the structure of the soft tissue. Looking at the back of a lean individual, we can see the outline of some of the superficial muscles that cover the back of the body. Figure 14 in the insert shows the overlapping layers of muscle. The top layer is the latissimus dorsi (lats).

At its lower end, and close to the spine and hip, it is covered by a silvery tissue, the thoracolumbar fascia. As we go deeper, we uncover other muscles that participate in keeping our spine erect and facilitating movement. All the muscles that support and move the spine can be a source of back pain, as can muscles not directly connected to the spine but that radiate pain to the muscles attached to the spine. Pain in the muscles of the back is often mistakenly assumed to be coming from the spine. Back discomfort may change the way we stand, sit, walk, run, and lift. We do this to make ourselves feel less distress without recognizing that over time, these well-meaning changes in posture may produce more muscle and connective tissue pain.

THE MUSCLES UNDER THE LATS

- The serratus posterior inferior (SPI), which is attached to the ribs and the thoracic spine, pulls down the ribs to create a larger cavity in the chest so that the lungs can expand more when we need extra oxygen for physically demanding situations such as running. Some patients may give me a clue that their midback pain is related to the SPI when they tell me that their pain is worse when they take a deep breath.

- The longissimus thoracis extends from your sacrum and hip bone up to almost all of your ribs and allows you to stand up straight. When only one side contracts, it allows you to bend to that side.

- The muscle adjacent to the longissimus is the iliocostalis lumborum, which is also attached to the sacrum and the top of the hip, and extends up to and attaches to the lower ribs, the thoracolumbar fascia, and the transverse processes of the upper lumbar vertebrae.

• The next layer down reveals both the quadratus lumborum, which attaches to the twelfth rib, close to the diaphragm (the muscle at the bottom of your rib cage that forces air in and out of your lungs when it contracts and relaxes), the lumbar spine, and top of the hip, and the multifidus muscle, which attaches to the sacrum and the lumbar spine.

• Abdominal muscles—yes, abdominal muscles can be a source of back pain because they attach to the hip bone at the outer edge of your back. Abdominal oblique muscles originate on the hip bone (on the iliac crest) and insert into the fascia surrounding the rectus abdominus, while the rectus abdominus muscles begin on the pubic symphysis (the spot where the two pubic bones join) and insert in four locations: the fifth to seventh ribs and the sternum, or breastbone.

  Your back pain can come from your abdominal muscles directly when one of them is a source of pain from an injury, or it may be related to muscle weakness, such as what happens as a result of childbirth. In fact, weak abdominal muscles are one of the most frequent reasons for failure of the Kraus-Weber test for trunk muscle strength and flexibility (which I will discuss in Chapter 9).

• The iliopsoas is composed of the iliacus, which is the muscle overlying the inner side of the hip bone, and the psoas major, which originates on the lumbar spines. Together these muscles insert into the femur (thigh bone) to flex and externally rotate the hip.

  The quadratus lumborum and psoas major sandwich a collection of nerves (the *lumbar plexus*) that exit the spinal cord in the lumbar spine. If either or both muscles are stiff, they can squeeze the lumbar plexus and cause pain and loss of sensation in the thigh and leg. This may be mistakenly interpreted as coming from nerve compression in the spine due to a bulging or herniated disc.

• The muscles in the buttocks also cause pain that may be reported as low back pain. Many of my patients, when they are showing me their low back pain, actually put their hand on their buttock. All the buttock muscles, which are involved in moving the hip, are frequently a source of low back and buttock pain. The largest muscle in the body, the gluteus maximus, is the most superficial of the buttock muscles. The deeper muscles are the gluteus medius, piriformis, gemellus, and obturator. All the muscles of the buttock and upper thigh are shown in figure 15 in the insert.

• The muscles of the thigh may cause leg pain, but they can also be a cause of low back and buttock pain. The leg muscles that I often find contribute to back pain are the adductor magnus and the hamstrings. However, the rectus femoris, vastus medialis, tensor fasciae latae, vastus lateralis, pectineus, gracilis, and sartorius may also play a role. See figure 16 in the insert for a visual representation of the thigh muscles.

Muscles can cause pain through three different mechanisms:

1. Directly from the injured muscle.

2. Nerve compression. Nerves may travel through or next to a muscle. If that muscle is tight and swollen, it can squeeze those nerves. Two areas where

this frequently occurs are the piriformis muscle and the region where the quadratus lumborum and psoas muscles overlap. The piriformis often surrounds the large sciatic nerve, while the quadratus and the psoas lie where nerves forming the lumbar plexus leave the spinal cord. If any of these muscles are too tight, the nerves may be squeezed, sending pain down the leg. A doctor may confuse this with pain coming from a nerve that's being compressed by a herniated disc. Since there is a good chance an imaging study will reveal problems with your spine, such as a degenerated or herniated disc, if the muscles aren't taken into account as a possible cause of the pain, the only treatment considered will be something to address the finding on the imaging study. That's one reason why epidural steroid injections, facet blocks, and surgeries frequently fail.

3. Referred pain from muscles, which can open inactive nerve pathways and cause pain to be experienced in an adjacent or distant, uninvolved muscle. More on this in Chapter 5.

MUSCLES OF THE MID AND UPPER BACK

The muscles of the midback and upper back (which can be seen in figure 17 in the insert) are sometimes involved in producing upper back pain and, at times, even lower back pain—particularly when the back pain is generalized rather than in a specific area. Some of the muscles already mentioned extend from the lower back to the upper back. Muscles that I often find to be important in the back of the chest are:

• Infraspinatus—the muscle that covers the lower part of your shoulder blade. It is the most common muscle to cause shoulder pain.

• Teres major—sits on the outside of the infraspinatus and is usually also a source of pain.

• Trapezius—where most of us feel the shoulder pain. However, at least half the time, I find that the pain actually comes from the infraspinatus and only refers to the trapezius.

The following are frequently sources of shoulder and neck pain:

• Rhomboids

• Levator scapula

• Serratus anterior

• Splenius capitis

• Subscapularis

• Teres minor

• Triceps

• Supraspinatus

On the front of the chest wall, the pectoralis major and minor, and the anterior, medial, and posterior scalenes muscles have all been found to contribute to upper back and neck pain. See figures 18 and 19 in the insert for an illustration of the neck, head, chest wall, and facial muscles.

For those of you who want to have more detailed knowledge of these muscles, you can refer to the atlases mentioned in the "Recommended Readings" section.

Muscles are layered one on top of another. Therefore, if your doctor or therapist presses on only one spot of your back, and it is tender, he or she can't know for certain which muscle in the layer is causing the pain. Both the origin and the point of insertion, or entheses, where the muscle connects to the tendon and the tendon attaches to the bone, contain the highest number of pain-sensitive nerves. Examining the muscle properly requires both the knowledge of muscle anatomy in the area of complaint and the expertise to examine their attachments. It may be difficult to feel the attachments, especially in deep muscles. Pressing to find the painful muscle has been a challenge to doctors ever since we first recognized that muscles could be the source of pain. In Chapter 19, I will introduce to you a revolutionary medical instrument that allows anyone examining you to know which muscle is causing your pain and why.

CHAPTER 5

Pain from Damage in Your Spine

What is a normal back?

You might be able to guess what the answer is.

If "normal" is defined as what we find in most people when we look at imaging studies, abnormal is normal. Most spines are not perfect, and the anatomical imperfection can be inappropriately labeled as "sick" (a pathology), but in truth, that's just a variation of "normal." Throughout our lives, wear and tear occurs in every part of our body. This is normal. If the wear and tear is extreme, it's a problem, but that still doesn't tell us that this problem is causing your pain. X-rays and MRIs of some terrible-looking spines are from people without pain complaints!

But can't we have any general description of a normal back? Yes. A normal, healthy back is reasonably aligned from top to bottom, with two natural curves (lordosis) in the neck and the low back (see figure 5). There is adequate distance between the vertebrae of the spine so that bone is not touching bone. The nerves and the spinal cord are not significantly compressed. The muscles that help hold us erect and produce proper posture are pliable, flexible, reasonably strong, and are able to sustain activity for a reasonable period of time (endurance). I realize this is not very specific, but it is an overview of what I, my colleague Hans Kraus, and his colleagues at Columbia University found in most of our patients who were able to become pain free.

If there is pain, it can be the result of more than one structure in the back: bones, nerves, cartilage, muscles, and other soft tissues such as tendons, ligaments, and fascia. How each of these contributes will be explored, but don't forget: muscles are the largest organ system by weight and are the major reason that any of us have back pain.

As with all parts of the body, the spine undergoes wear and tear, called *spondylosis* or *spinal osteoarthritis*. The discs lose water and become flatter. It's called degenerative disc disease (DDD), but it isn't a disease—it's just what happens as we get older. It is why people become shorter with age. We can see DDD and spondylosis on an X-ray, but it is not usually the reason for your pain. Figure 20 in the insert shows a degenerated, flattened disc.

The spinal problem that people most commonly hear about and fear is a herniated disc, frequently called a slipped disc by nonmedical people. This occurs when wear or an injury opens a tear in the ligament surrounding your disc and a piece of it pops out. Sometimes the ligament can stretch and not tear. It would be seen on an imaging study as a bulging disc. This happens so often in patients who do not experience pain that most physicians no longer feel that it is a significant finding. Actually, even patients with a herniated disc may have no pain at all, while others do. On occasion, surgery may be necessary to deal with back pain, but not when the pain originates in muscle tissue. To repeat the mantra yet again, *the primary source of 75 percent or more of all back pain is from the muscles, not the spine.*

Certainly there are instances when surgery for a herniated disc is helpful and even dramatically necessary. For example, surgery should be considered when the protruding jellylike material squeezes a nerve in your back that causes pain to run from the buttock, down the leg, to the foot, and to the toes, and if in addition, you complain of diminished reflexes, loss of sensation, weakness, and shrinkage of the painful muscles, along with a lack of control of your urinary and anal sphincters. Similarly, surgery should be taken into consideration when the jellylike material presses upon a nerve in your neck, causing pain in your arm and fingers as well as the same set of associated symptoms. In both instances, an operation known as *decompressive foraminotomy* or *decompressive laminectomy* can solve the problem and end the pain. In decompressive foraminotomy, portions of the vertebra may be removed to widen the foramen (the hole in the vertebra) and thus decompress a nerve root (the part of the nerve first exiting the spinal cord—see figure 12). Decompressive laminectomy, on the other hand, removes part of the vertebra (the lamina) and sometimes thickened connective tissue that both narrow the spinal canal and squeeze the nerve roots and spinal cord. See figure 13.

Fortunately, we see very few patients who have such clear-cut indications for surgery. Even when there is a herniated disc, and some of these signs and symptoms are found, surgery may not successfully relieve the pain. Remember, the commonly held belief that damaged discs are the fundamental cause of most low back pain is mistaken. Many disc surgeries are failures, as measured by the fact that patients experience no improvement or may even suffer increased back pain. The number of unsuccessful back surgeries has soared so high that a new diagnosis was created based on the persistence of pain and other symptoms postsurgery—something unique in all of medicine—called *failed back surgery syndrome* (FBSS). It is also known as postlaminectomy syndrome because it refers to the part of the vertebra, the lamina, that is cut away to remove pressure from the squeezed nerve.

Persistent pain can also develop when the spinal column is unstable. If the vertebrae do not lie cleanly on top of one another because of slippage, known as spondylolisthesis, they can painfully move back and forth when you're in motion. See figure 21 in the insert for an illustration of this.

If the depth of a vertebra is two inches, and one vertebra sits at least one inch beyond the vertebra above or below, we would consider this significant spondylolisthesis. If that's the case, the patient might benefit from spinal fusion, which eliminates the movement between vertebrae that may be causing the pain. If the movement is between L3 and L4, and L4 and L5, then L3, L4, and L5 would be fused together by inserting a rod with hooks into the bone, taking extra bone harvested from the hip or from a bone donor bank and layering it between the vertebrae. The patient would then have one solid bone from L3 to L5, minimizing motion in the spine and possibly eliminating the pain. One difficulty is that the small movement demonstrated on an X-ray may not be the cause of the pain, and so eliminating the motion may not eliminate the pain. In addition, if the spine can't move in one area, it will have to move more in the segments above and below the fusion. These segments will then undergo more wear and tear, and, if it becomes serious enough, the patient may need additional fusion.

Failed spinal surgery is a growing problem. It consigns a patient to an increasing population composed of people who believe that they are destined to suffer persistent pain for the rest of their lives. Generally, they have two common options for some relief:

1. *Spinal cord stimulator:* a small electrical-impulse generator that is placed surgically under your skin with wires leading from it to the tissue around the spinal cord. The electrical impulses can mask the pain signals, providing some relief.

2. Strong pain medication, such as morphine-like drugs, and sometimes with it antispasm medication, taken orally or through a pump that deposits the medication to the area around the spinal cord.

We have been successful in eliminating pain in many failed back surgery patients, even after multiple failed operations, by identifying muscles that were always the reason for the pain. (See Chapter 19.) And now an increasing number of clinicians, including orthopedic surgeons and neurosurgeons, recognize that the problem of back pain is more complex than what might seem to be apparent in images of the discs, joints, and nerves of the spine. They realize that many factors, such as emotional stress, job issues, and physical conditioning, all contribute to back pain.

Still, although back pain abounds on an epidemic scale, it remains a puzzle to too many doctors. One reason is that they do not believe that the main cause of back pain is sprains and strains of soft tissue, primarily muscles. Instead they believe that if muscle pain exists at all, it is only as a result of irritated or compressed nerves. Sometimes this can be the case, but it is definitely not true for the overwhelming majority of patients with back pain. Their distress is caused by physical and chemical changes in muscle tissue, a subject dealt with at length in Chapter 6.

CENTRAL SENSITIZATION (CS) AND DIFFUSE NOXIOUS INHIBITORY CONTROL (DNIC)

A problem in understanding back pain is related to two conflicting mechanisms in the nervous system. One is *central sensitization*; the other is *diffuse noxious inhibitory control*, now called *conditioned pain modulation* (CPM).

When the muscles send painful impulses to the nerves, the nerves transmit that information to the spinal cord, which becomes excited electrically. This increased spinal cord activity—central sensitization (CS)—is like turning up the volume on your DVD player before putting on the disc. When you press Play, it sounds way too loud. The same thing happens in your body: there is too much response for the amount of input, which leads you to experience pain even though you didn't do anything that would normally hurt. Something else happens in CS: the pain spreads to muscles not involved in the activity that spurred the pain. This is called *referred pain.* Referred pain can also come from a joint, i.e. an arthritic hip can cause knee pain; myocardial infarction, commonly called a heart attack, can cause chest wall or arm pain. Sometimes just by eliminating or easing the worst pain—generally in the muscle area where the pain began— the pain in the other muscle areas disappears.

This happened to a patient we'll call Roberta, who suffered from back, neck, shoulder, and headache pain after her car was rear-ended. She saw a neurologist, a neurosurgeon, and an orthopedic surgeon, all of whom agreed that a noninvasive intervention, physical therapy, should be tried first. Unable to do the exercises or the stretching because she felt worse afterward, the surgeons then suggested spinal fusion. Roberta was fearful of surgery. She eventually took a cocktail of pain medications that included oxycodone, the anticonvulsant pregabalin, and the antidepressant duloxetine. Yet nothing relieved the pain.

After spending weeks in bed, she was in despair, unable to get up to care for her two teenage daughters or to perform her usual chores around the house. On the advice of a friend, whom I had treated, she came to me for a consultation. I found thirteen muscles in her upper and lower body that appeared to be the cause of her pain. I began by treating her worst pain, which was in the neck and upper back. But after treating five of the muscles to relieve her upper body pain, all the pain in her lower back also disappeared. In other words, the pain in her upper back and neck and headache had caused CS of her spinal cord. The pain had spread to her lower body. Treating the upper body muscles was all that her condition required.

Just as CS causes you to feel more pain, CPM causes you to feel less pain. You may have experienced something like this: you feel pain in your toe, and then you develop a blinding headache. Suddenly you forget the toe because of the more severe headache.

When CPM and CS occur simultaneously, confusion can occur. The case history of a patient whom I shall call Jerry, a forty-year-old carpenter, is a good example.

For years, Jerry felt pain in his right shoulder, and he had seen many doctors. Some said that thinning spinal discs in his neck were the cause and suggested nerve blocks. One doctor even urged a cervical (neck) fusion. Others thought that Jerry's pain was broadcasting from the trapezius muscle on top of the shoulder.

When I examined him, the only tender muscle in his shoulder was over the shoulder blade—not the trapezius but a different one, the infraspinatus. However, when treatment relieved the pain in the infraspinatus, a reexamination found that *another* muscle, the rhomboid, had become painful. Treating that muscle totally eliminated Jerry's shoulder pain.

His case makes it evident that diagnosing pain may not be a simple matter. Indeed, the apparent reason for a particular pain may change as treatment progresses. Frequent reevaluation is important to determine whether a suspect muscle is still painful or a previously tested pain-free muscle has become a new pain generator.

Imagine if your pain has been present for more than ten years. An initial, even minor injury can cause pain to be covered over by layers of new pain in other areas of your body. The mechanisms that caused the original pain may continue to operate, but you're not conscious of the original discomfort. This happened with a patient I shall call Lenore. Her pain began in her legs when she was ten years old. It spread progressively into her whole body, until pain became the center of her life. It interfered with her ability to think, sleep, and do all physical activities. She was diagnosed with fibromyalgia, as are many patients with total body pain. Lenore wrote the following after six months of treatment with me:

As I near the age of 25, I am finally beginning to physically feel like my real chronological age as opposed to the 80-year-old woman I have felt like for the past 15 years of my life. Before the age of 10, I was a "normal," active young girl who played tennis, went to sleepaway camp, and didn't have to think twice about playing games like tag or sports with my friends. That all began to change as I experienced intense pain in my legs while at overnight camp that would not go away. On November 4, 1997, I was diagnosed with fibromyalgia, an illness that would affect every aspect of my life. I was in constant 24-hour chronic pain, unable to stay awake most of the day, yet found it impossible to sleep at night. Because of fibromyalgia, my mind was almost always a blank, making it difficult to concentrate and hold a long conversation.

Two out of my four years of high school, I was placed on home instruction and was unable to physically make it to school. This had a negative impact on my social life. In addition to all the physical effects this illness had on me, the toll it took on my emotional health was astronomical as well. I was in a deep depression and did not really see much of a way out. I completed my under-graduate and graduate degrees, but my pain only continued to worsen. The mere thought of this pain being a part of my everyday existence drastically increased my depression.

The summer before I met Dr. Marcus, I was on vacation and needed to use a wheelchair for the whole two weeks. By the time I went to Dr. Marcus for my initial consultation, I had practically given up hope. After going to so many doctors and trying so many different treatments, there is only so much disappointment one can take.

Through all my years of living with fibromyalgia, no doctor has ever tried to specifically treat the muscles. Fibromyalgia is believed to be an illness of the central nervous system, and most doctors try to treat the symptoms (pain, fatigue, insomnia) through medication, diet, and exercise, but don't actually treat the source of the pain. For me, treating the symptoms never worked.

During my initial evaluation, I was not able to specify where the pain was; I described it as "everywhere." While being examined by Dr. Marcus, it became evident that although I felt the pain throughout my entire body, not every muscle in my body was causing pain. Once the treatments began and the pain in certain muscles began to disappear, I was able to identify specific areas on my body that were in pain, as opposed to that overwhelming pain I felt "everywhere" during that initial evaluation.

After 6 months of treatment with Dr. Marcus, I can honestly say I feel like a new person. A month into treatment, I was able to walk a mile for the first time in 15 years. I am beginning to look for a job, get off some of my depression medication, decrease my dosage of pain medication, and have a whole new outlook on life. I finally see a bright, exciting future filled with endless possibilities, as opposed to a future filled with daily physical pain and depression.

CHAPTER 6

Muscles and Back Pain

Muscles need to be strong and flexible and have adequate endurance to perform an activity for the time required. You could have the strength to lift fifty pounds, but you may not have the endurance to hold it for three minutes. No matter what your strength or endurance, the task you are asked to do may be damaging over time because of the repetitive nature of the activity.

One of the most interesting patients I have seen was a pastry chef at a well-known New York restaurant. Pain in her low back and buttock radiated down her thigh and calf, and produced some tingling in her toes. At first it sounded as if her sciatic nerve was being compressed, but the chef's examination did not reveal any loss of sensation, weakness, or reflex changes—in other words, no other red flags. She did have tenderness in her buttock, but it was mostly in one muscle, the piriformis (see figure 22 in the insert). It attaches to the greater trochanter, a bony protuberance on the thigh bone (femur), and also to the lower portion of the spine (the sacrum).

Contracting the piriformis pulls the femur, causing outward rotation of the hip and movement of the thigh away from the center of the body. Up until then,

I had only seen patients with a painful piriformis who also had other painful muscles in their buttock and/or low back. She didn't. I couldn't understand how this happened until I took a very detailed account of what the chef did at work. She told me she rolled dough on a marble slab, cut it into small pieces for her pastries, and placed them on a tray. After opening the oven door, which was below her work table, she bent down to place the baking tray on a shelf in the oven, and as she stood up, she placed the side of her shoe under the oven door, energetically lifting it to slam it shut. I asked her how many times a day she did this, and she said more than fifteen!

Case solved. It is always important to discover what activities may be the source of the pain, so that each patient can change his or her habits and eliminate future recurrences of pain.

The pastry chef was lucky, as she came to see me soon after the pain began. She was able to eliminate her pain in two weeks by using her hand rather than her foot to close the oven door, along with electrical stimulation and massage to relax her stiffened muscle. Can you think of any activity that you do at home, in the office, or during play that might be straining muscles and contributing to your pain?

This case demonstrates another interesting fact about back pain. Relatively few nerve cells represent the back and the buttock, which often makes it difficult for pain sufferers to pinpoint exactly where they hurt. A pain in the low back could be experienced as being in the buttock and vice versa. The piriformis caused pain in the low back and buttock. A physician should conduct a thorough examination of all the muscles that could be contributing to the pain in order to narrow down which muscle and physical movements could be the culprits.

MUSCLE FACTS

Back problems can be very misunderstood and costly. Treatments rely far too often on expensive surgery, lifelong use of potent medications, and other widely used interventions such as nerve blocks and stimulators to "manage" pain rather than eliminate it altogether. The doctors who provide this treatment mean well. They *want* to help you. But they are victims of the system almost as much as you are. I, too, was misguided, as I mentioned earlier, when I relied on teaching patients in my multidisciplinary pain program to live with their pain instead of properly diagnosing and treating the muscles that caused it. Although I still believe that some pain patients are best managed in a multidisciplinary setting, I know now that most of them can have their pain relieved.

Hans once said to me, "If you asked your patients would they prefer to manage or eliminate their pain, what do you think they would say?" The answer was obvious. Good intentions are no excuse for not treating the cause of the pain.

A considerable part of the problem lies in medical education. At best, muscle pain is given short shrift in medical school and is usually missing in the mainstream literature on pain treatment. Scientists have always had difficulty understanding how muscles cause pain. It has been clear that muscles may be tender to pressure, but the reason for the tenderness and finding effective treatment have been elusive. You won't find any discussion of muscle pain in any major medical textbook on comprehensive pain treatment. Specialized books on muscle pain will address the subject, of course, but it is not generally included in the curricula for medical students or for physicians who specialize in pain treatment and management. It is as if basic dentistry texts made no mention of cavities. This will change in 2012 with the publication of two major pain management textbooks, which will contain chapters on muscle pain.

What doctors *will* find in any comprehensive textbook on pain is a chapter on *myofascial pain syndrome* (MPS). MPS is pain related to the muscles (myo) and connective tissue (fascia), which refers to fascia, tendons, and ligaments. The term, however, is not used consistently. Doctors frequently—and mistakenly—use *myofascial pain* and *myofascial trigger point* interchangeably. As I explain below, a myofascial trigger point is only one of four major reasons for common muscle pain. Even the International Association for the Study of Pain, in describing muscle pain in its suggested core curriculum for physicians, reports that myofascial pain "lacks reliable means for physicians to identify, categorize, and treat such pain." That means there is no standard protocol.

Even the terminology has been ill-defined and confusing since the sixteenth century. Our medical ancestors knew that muscles were causing pain, but just like us, they couldn't figure out how it happened or what the treatment should be. The various names they gave to muscle pain reflect this confusion. Some of the terms that have been used over the years are *myitis, muscular rheumatism, myalgia, myogelosen, Muskelhärten, fibrositis,* and *myofibrositis*.

Fibromyalgia syndrome (FMS) is a current example. FMS is characterized by chronic pain throughout the body. Other symptoms may include stiffness in the joints, excessive sensitivity to pressure, inability to sleep, and extreme fatigue.

Current medical thinking regards FMS as a problem in the nervous system—perhaps increased activity in the spinal cord—that makes a person too susceptible to stimuli. But recent studies have shown that the muscles in patients diagnosed with FMS can be the significant pain generators. Furthermore, as with my patient Lenore, if the muscle pain is diminished, some or all of the FMS symptoms will be alleviated too.

It is not surprising that back pain patients are confused. Let's end the confusion. I want you to understand the science so that you can have the knowledge and peace of mind to take the first step toward recovery.

When scientists and doctors talk about the cause of a problem, such as pain in the body, they use the term *pathophysiological mechanism*. In this case, it means the process that produces pain in muscle tissue. Here's how it works: a series of chain reactions, so to speak, starts with three different types of nerves known as muscle nociceptors. These nerves are sensitive to changes that occur when you damage a muscle or are in danger of damaging it: for example, through repeated overuse or by trying to lift more than your muscle can bear.

The two different nerve types that have been identified in muscle are:

1. *High-threshold mechanoreceptors*, which are sensitive to excessive pressure, such as when a muscle is squeezed tightly or punched.

2. *Polymodal nociceptors*, which are sensitive to both chemical and mechanical stimulation.

When tissue is damaged, it releases chemicals that stimulate these nerve receptors. (Even a muscle strain may be enough to release these chemicals.) The stimulated nerves, in turn, release a variety of additional chemicals, which collectively include Substance P, calcitonin gene-related peptide, somatostatin, bradykinin, histamine, and adenosine triphosphate (ATP). These make up what is sometimes called a vasoneuroactive "soup." This soup causes the small blood vessels to leak blood fluid, called plasma, into the localized area of damaged muscle tissue. That may result in swelling, which squeezes the blood vessels that bring blood and oxygen to the injured area. If the tissue does not heal properly, the reduced oxygen and accumulated chemical soup may contribute to the formation of what is called a trigger point.

If that happens, the muscle is changed and may not recover unless treatment to break up the nodule is initiated. Untreated, this area of swollen tissue squeezes the small blood vessels and reduces both the blood flow and the oxygen supply to the muscle. The condition can last for years and could be the reason for continuing back pain.

Once the nerves in the muscle are stimulated, they send signals to the spinal cord and stimulate cells there. In turn, these nerves in the spinal cord send signals to the brain, as if shouting "Look out!" as a warning to respond, either to prevent injury or to minimize the damage that already has occurred.

These stimulated spinal cord nerves do something else very interesting and very pertinent: they open up closed connections both higher up and lower down in the spinal cord, exciting them, too. This can make you experience pain in these areas as well. It is called *referred pain* because your body is telling you that you have pain, say, in your buttock or your neck, when the sensation is actually coming from muscles in your low back or shoulder.

When the nerves are stimulated for too long a period of time, they become sensitized; in other words, they react more to stimuli. An example would be a physical movement that you previously could do comfortably or with minimal discomfort but now causes you pain. We call this response *muscle allodynia* (pain from a movement that is typically not painful) or *hyperalgesia* (more pain than you typically experience from a pain-inducing event).

Another change happens when nerves are sensitized: pressure on an area is felt as tenderness rather than the sensation of being strongly touched. If damage to muscle tissue goes undetected, all of this can continue for weeks, months, years, even decades.

The entire muscle pain process is complex, as you can see. But the facts concerning the mechanisms that cause muscle pain are now available for anyone to read in the scientific literature.

Much of the fundamental research on muscle nerves and pain has come from the tireless work of Professor Siegfried Mense of the University of Heidelberg. He has enabled pain clinicians to understand how muscle pain is generated. His solid scientific evidence explains how back pain originates in muscles, no matter what was found on imaging studies. Thus, if a doctor tells you that your pain can come only from your spine or nerves, you will know better.

COMMON REASONS FOR MUSCLE PAIN CAUSED BY MISUSE (FUNCTIONAL MUSCLE PAIN)

Functional causes of muscle pain are causes having to do with the proper conditioning and usage of a muscle in contrast to the actual disease of a muscle (for example, muscular dystrophy). Putting aside the complicated chain reactions that produce muscle pain, let's look at what may happen in your life to make a muscle painful. Apart from muscle diseases, which are very rare, there are four different "functional causes" for any muscle pain: *tension, deficiency* (stiffness and/or weakness), *spasm,* and, as noted previously, trigger points. This chapter looks at muscle spasm and muscle deficiency. Chapter 7 examines tension, and Chapter 19, trigger points.

MUSCLE SPASM

A thirty-six-year-old patient I shall call Ellie came to me bent over in severe pain three months after the birth of her first child. She had not exercised at all for at least a year. She told me that she was determined to "knock off the weight" she had gained and "get back into shape." Ellie was so determined that she hit the gym for ten consecutive days, doing forty-five minutes each of spinning, running on the treadmill, and weight lifting each day. She felt some stiffness in her right low back but believed that it came with the territory of a newly inspired gym warrior. But one morning when she awoke, her back pain and stiffness were so severe that she could barely get out of bed. Movement in any direction was excruciating; bending over was out of the question. The pain was focused in her low back and the top of her buttock. She was terrified, fearful that she had ruptured a disc. I saw her the same day.

Muscle spasm is unmistakable. It can strike anytime after you suffer an acute sprain, strain, or fracture, and it can come seemingly out of nowhere. It may be brought on simply by sneezing or getting out of bed; crouching to pick up something; lifting; shoveling snow; or any number of ordinary activities. Low back spasm can be excruciating. You can't stand up straight, one hip is higher than the other—you are literally "bent out of shape." If you try to move, the pain shoots across your back like a ceaseless electric shock.

The crippling pain can last for hours; days even, if the spasm is not broken. Suddenly, however—without having done anything for it—the spasm will vanish, as if it never happened. Yet it is likely to seize you again when you least expect it. Sometimes just wondering whether it might return can bring it back with a surge. Indeed, when a back spasm strikes, it can be so wrenching that you may very well think you've been injured permanently. Don't panic. Back spasm does not have to signify a serious condition, and it is highly likely that it stems from your muscles and it will get better.

A friend or family member can help interrupt the spasm by applying an ice pack to the painful area until it is numb. Do not leave it on too long though or you can get ice burn. Then gently move your back. As the pain subsides, slowly increase the movement until you are approaching your normal range of motion. Do this gently. Do not force the movement. Although most people will respond to the ice pack, if it doesn't provide relief, a hot pack or a series of hot towels applied to your back may help diminish the pain sufficiently for you to start moving gently so as to break the spasm.

In Ellie's case, an examination did not show any signs of serious problems or of nerve compression, such as pain down her leg, loss of sensation or tingling down her leg, or true weakness. I use the term "true weakness" because you may not be able to strongly contract painful muscles, giving the false appearance of weakness. This type of weakness is called *pain inhibition*. When that same muscle is not experiencing pain, a strong contraction is possible. With actual damage to the muscle or the nerve serving the muscle, maximally strong contraction is never possible.

The muscles in Ellie's right low back were hard and tender. I told her that she had a spasm and that our protocol was to provide two types of muscle stimulation with ice applied to the area: ten minutes of a continuous contraction (tetanizing), followed by ten minutes of a rhythmic contraction, and then doing the first seven exercises for low back pain outlined in Chapter 10.

Ellie felt better after each session, and after four consecutive days of treatment, her spasm was totally gone. She was then given the additional low back exercises comprising the full regimen of Kraus-Marcus exercises for low back pain. We also went over the concepts associated with proper training, which is especially important when you have not been exercising for a long time: begin slowly; add exercises and increase the difficulty and amount of time you exercise in small increments; and do not go to the next level until you are comfortable at your current level for at least one week.

MUSCLE DEFICIENCY

Two patients go to see their doctor for back pain. They have no signs that their pain originates in the spine. It seems to be coming from the muscles. One patient is overweight and never exercises or goes to the gym. The other is trim and exercises regularly. To understand why both of them can have pain originating in their muscles, we need to understand what makes a healthy muscle.

Muscle deficiency is simply defined as stiffness and/or weakness. This condition occurs when we do not get enough proper exercise. The overall problem is often referred to as deconditioning. Proper exercise begins first by relaxing so as to ease the physical tension in the muscles, then by limbering (movement through the range of comfort of the muscle being exercised) in order to gently diminish stiffness. This is followed by stretching to further overcome stiffness, and, finally, by strengthening.

Muscle stiffness prevents full range of motion of a muscle. If you have been using your muscles in an unhealthy way—let's say that you never stretch your back or thigh muscles—chances are that you can't touch your toes when bending at the waist with your knees kept straight. The reason is that your muscles are stiff. Similarly, if you've rarely held an outstretched arm up above your head, you may feel stiffness and resistance in the arm and shoulder muscles when trying to do so.

Many muscle exercises emphasize strength, but strength is only one characteristic of healthy muscles. If you are very strong yet very stiff, you do not have healthy muscles. You may look good, but a muscle-bound body doesn't work well. Healthy muscles are relaxed. Movement through a complete range should be easy, without pain. Healthy movement is graceful. Healthy muscles work fluidly, from relatively complete shortening contraction to relatively complete lengthening extension. And they are strong enough to accomplish specific tasks.

Healthy muscles are the product of proper physical activity and exercise best begun in childhood and continued into adulthood. But it is never too late to begin. Be aware, however, that even if you are athletic, you can still overdo strength at the expense of flexibility—and it is often more difficult to overcome stiffness than to overcome weakness.

Consider the twenty-eight-year-old runner who, after completing two marathons, came to see me, complaining of low back pain. An examination showed that he had normal X-rays and MRIs and sufficient strength. His problem was stiffness in his hamstrings, calf muscles, and low back. From a standing position, he could raise a straight leg only 40 degrees, when normal range of motion is at least 75 degrees; and when bending from the waist without bending his knees, he could come within only eighteen inches of touching his toes with his fingers.

I corrected his workout routine so that it included warming up and cooling down, with stretching. I had him cut back on all weight training for his legs, because strengthening a stiff muscle only makes it stiffer. I also had him cut back on running and instead had him take fast, long walks, coupled with a prescribed stretching program. Once his flexibility returned, he would be able to resume running.

But couch potatoes with back pain are the star exhibits of muscle deficiency, because they have *both* stiff and weak muscles. Any ordinary reaching or stretching can bring on gasps, grunts, and pain. Their combination of weak and stiff muscles is an open invitation to injury. A couch potato's muscles are like old rubber bands—stiff and ready to snap. And the longer he avoids exercise, the more deconditioned he becomes as more simple movements become uncomfortable. As the list of uncomfortable activities increases, life's possibilities shrink. Even if you are not a couch potato, you may associate pain with various things you do in your daily life and end up avoiding those things—walking, bicycling, stretching—the list goes on. This is called *kinesiophobia,* which is the avoidance of activity because you fear it will cause pain. If you are recovering from a painful episode, you will have to wisely overcome your fear of movement. You can get a sense of how your fear of injuring yourself is contributing to your problem's functioning by taking the Tampa Scale for Kinesiophobia, which you can find online at http://bit.ly/xWQBpe. The higher the score, the more fear is interfering with your ability to get better.

Loss of strength and muscle mass occurs as we age, thanks in part to inactivity. An extreme, but not unusual example, is weakness resulting from bed rest during illness or after an accident or surgery. Complete bed rest heightens all the negatives of inactivity. The dramatic change that accompanies complete bed rest has been termed the "disuse syndrome." A person can lose 1 percent to 3 percent of muscle strength for every day of bed rest. Thus, two weeks in bed can result in a nearly 40 percent loss of muscle strength with a simultaneous stiffening of the muscles.

Neither ice nor heat nor tranquilizers will do any good for muscle deficiency. But the twenty-one exercises explained and illustrated in Chapter 10 will do a world of good. They were developed specifically to correct muscle weakness and stiffness, and, as an added bonus, to teach relaxation skills, which all of us, young and old alike, can use.

CHAPTER 7

Stress, Tension, and Pain

Before you begin this chapter, please write down whatever thoughts come to your mind when you think about your pain. If you are not sure what I mean, it may help to complete the following phrases:

My pain is . . .

I have pain because . . .

My pain means . . .

Take at least five minutes to do this. As you keep thinking, some thoughts may occur that are not immediately apparent. After the five minutes are up, keep your notes handy. We are going to refer to them.

Unlike muscle stiffness, muscle tension comes from a voluntary contraction of a muscle. Our muscles sometimes contract when we are uncomfortable emotionally. Do you grit your teeth when you are angry? Do you notice that your neck and shoulders tighten when you are anxious about making a deadline? Is your back pain worse when you are fearful or resentful? All of these feelings may be put into a single category: mental stress.

It's important to recognize that thoughts and feelings travel to your muscles and can bring about low back pain, neck pain, and a throbbing tension headache. There is medical wisdom in common sayings such as "She is a pain in the neck" or "He gives me a headache." We all have people we love to hate. Whoever these tormentors are, they are living in your head rent free.

What you may not realize, however, is that negative thoughts may actually exacerbate the pain. Functional MRI (fMRI) can measure the metabolic activity (for example, how much glucose is consumed) in different areas of the brain. fMRI studies of pain sufferers demonstrate that negative thoughts can excite areas of the brain associated with pain perceptions and can intensify the sensation of pain.

Here is a simple exercise that will help you understand how the mind-muscle connection works. I want you to recall an unhappy incident in which someone important to you disappointed you or left you feeling hurt and angry. Think about that incident and how upset you were.

Now look in the mirror at the expression on your face. Try to exaggerate the expression. Make fists and grit your teeth. Tighten your shoulder muscles. Can you see your anger? What does it feel like? Is there an effect on your back pain? Most of you are likely to feel an increase in your pain.

Studies have shown that nonpainful muscles become tense during times of stress but quickly relax when the stress disappears. This is not the case with painful muscles, which remain contracted and tight long past the thought or feeling that set them off. What's interesting is that you don't have to feel intensely upset for stress to produce pain in your muscles. If you were to imagine feeling only a small percentage of the stress that you felt during the exercise—say, 25 percent of it—that would still be enough to affect your muscles and cause you some pain.

Now that you are aware that uncomfortable thoughts and feelings can increase your pain, it would be wonderful to stop the negative chatter in your mind. But that's easier said than done. As hard as it is to change those things we don't like about ourselves, it is much worse when we cannot even admit that we have thoughts and feelings that we regard as unacceptable. Denying that we have unacceptable thoughts has been shown to be not only ineffective but also physically harmful. For example, the denial of stressful feelings increases heart rate and blood pressure. It can't be repeated enough: if you have unconscious anxieties and resentments, muscle tension increases and pain worsens.

Breathing and stress are also linked. One of the ways that we suppress our feelings is by holding our breath. Observe yourself when you are nervous. Notice that your breathing is shallow. Whenever you feel threatened, emotionally or otherwise, your breathing is generally shallower than usual. This too contributes to increased muscle pain. Sufficient oxygen is required for normal muscle function. When a muscle is deprived of oxygen, it hurts.

It's strange that we humans want to be perfect and have such a hard time admitting that we're not. We all have thoughts and feelings that we don't like having. Recognizing them actually makes it less likely that you will act on them. Even so, acknowledging them in yourself requires the courage to be truthful with yourself. To do that, it sometimes helps to talk to someone you trust: a friend, spouse, therapist, or religious adviser. But the first step in dealing with these hidden thoughts and feelings, however you do it, is to recognize them.

Very recently, I had a patient whose recovery from chronic back pain I attribute partly to her willingness to face her demons. I will call her Marci, a forty-five-year-old Arizona housewife and mother of two teenagers. She was active in sports, very involved with her children in school functions, and very happy in her marriage.

Marci was moving furniture at home when she felt a sudden knife-like pain in her low back and buttock. The pain was incapacitating. She spent weeks in bed, and saw two surgeons, a neurologist, a physiatrist, and a couple of physical therapists. Individually and collectively, they informed her that she had minimal disc herniations that required a laminectomy, a spinal operation to remove a section of the vertebral bone called the lamina.

Instead of having the surgery, Marci came to see me at my practice in New York. During treatment, she told me that her pain always worsened whenever she was around her father or when she thought about him. They had never gotten along, and she had vowed that she would never be anything like him. As we spoke about him, she became angry. She thought of vivid, disappointing memories of family events. She began to cry. She talked about her feeling of emptiness and longing. She said that she had never gotten her father's support and probably never would. As we spoke, she began to realize that he too had come from an unsupportive home.

It took courage for Marci to reveal her feelings to me, something most troubled patients do not do so quickly, if at all. After the first week of treatment, most of her pain was eliminated. As she admitted her painful feelings, much of her generalized physical pain decreased while, at the same time, she became more aware of specific muscles where she felt most of her pain. She needed injections into some of them, but a reexamination showed that the painful muscles that I had not treated were no longer painful. This was no miracle. Marci's recovery occurred, as I've said, in part because the issues causing her stress even before her back pain occurred were so openly acknowledged and addressed.

Pain is not a condition that you are programmed to endure. Pain is not supposed to go on forever. Whenever you suffer some form of injury, your body generally heals in about six weeks. You feel better. But when the pain persists, chronic back pain especially, you wonder if you'll ever feel better. If you've suffered from back pain for longer than three months, chances are that you've had an X-ray, MRI, or CT scan that showed something wrong. Even if your pain eases or goes away for a time, you now believe you'll never be "normal" again. You become more cautious. You eliminate activities. You start to think you are getting old. You become wrapped up in the pain you have now or in the pain that you know you will have soon.

One of my patients, Allison, was immersed in her pain and unable to think of anything else. She was referred to me because both her gynecologist and her pain management physician thought that her complaints of back pain might be coming from muscles.

Allison had a long, complicated history. She was very active working as a computer designer, traveling to trade shows and working long hours. She was the center of her family, a confidante to her sisters and brother, and always in touch with her parents. She had loads of friends and was in love with her boyfriend. Then out of nowhere, she developed pain in her pelvis. Her gynecologist examined her and couldn't find any obvious problem. Her pain got worse, and she started to miss days of work, something she had never done and couldn't bear to do. The decision was made to perform a laparoscopy in her pelvis. In this procedure, a small tube with a lens is inserted into the abdominal/pelvic area, allowing the doctor to look inside while being minimally invasive. Nothing abnormal was seen. Her diagnosis—pelvic pain without pathology—is the same diagnosis that 33 percent of women with pelvic pain receive.

Allison's pelvic pain continued, but then it also moved into her low back and soon down her left leg to her knee. She was referred to a pain center. Because the back pain was radiating to her leg and disrupting her life, an MRI of her low back was done. It showed a small herniated disc in her lumbar spine. She received the usual treatment—an epidural steroid injection, which involved placing a small amount of a cortisone-like substance close to the compressed nerve in the spine that was thought to be causing the pain to radiate down the leg. She reported that she felt a little better for a week, and then the pain returned. Her pain doctor had found tender muscles in the areas where she complained of the pain, and after discussion with her gynecologist, he referred her to me.

Allison looked very sad and told me that she didn't know how she could go on with her life if the pain wasn't relieved. Although her pain was relentless, it fluctuated. When she was feeling better, she would test the pain by bending and twisting until she felt a twinge, and then she knew it was only a matter of time until it would attack her again full force.

You may find similarities in your life that remind you of Allison. She admitted, with embarrassment, that she wished she were dead at times, but being Catholic, she would never do anything to harm herself. I examined her, and, as I have found in so many patients, she had areas of muscle tenderness that seemed to come from tension. There were other areas too where it appeared that the muscle was altered and would benefit from injections. Since tension, weakness, and stiffness were major factors in her pain, I thought certain exercises would also help. She was taught the first two levels of the exercises you will learn in Chapter 10.

Allison's pain soon diminished, but, strangely, her mood got worse. She told me that she couldn't stop crying and didn't understand what was going on in her life.

It was terrible that for two years she lived in chronic pain. But losing her sense of identity as a hard-driving, productive worker and an important member of her family added to her suffering.

When people with back pain feel a twinge, it's easy for them to sink into a mood of self-defeat. "I can't take it!" "What did I do to deserve this?" "What's the use?" "I might as well be dead!" We pain physicians have a word for the self-destructive thoughts that make your pain worse and destroy your life. It's called "catastrophizing." Even if you had been a positive thinker with a zest for life before your chronic pain took hold, it's now a struggle to remember your optimism and joy.

There are many sayings about adversity. The nineteenth-century German philosopher Friedrich Nietzsche said, "What doesn't kill you makes you stronger." In the Bible, Corinthians tells us that God will not let you be tested beyond your strength. My favorite is one that Hans taught me: *Non tutti i mali vengono per nuocere*, which roughly translates to "every cloud has a silver lining."

One of the keys to your recovery is to overcome negative thinking. The best exercises, injections, pills, and massage cannot make you better when you believe you'll never be normal again. If pain becomes the dominant force in your life, you have let it destroy everything that used to be important to you. The following figure illustrates how pain can dominate your life.

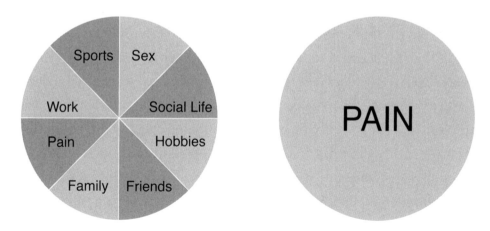

I promise you that you can get better and your life can improve, provided that you look closely at where you are, where you were, and where you want to be. I'm not saying you'll be able to ski the hardest trails again. You may not. But there are so many things that you will be able to do again that will bring pleasure back into your life.

Patients have said to me, "I can't help the way I feel!" Please remember, how we think *determines* how we feel. Negative thinking creates a negative response to events. How would you respond when asked about your pain? Would you say it feels "sharp and intense" or "killing and torturing"? Both statements may be applied to the same pain, but one describes sensation, and the other describes suffering. Studies show that patients who say they are "tortured" by pain function less well in their daily activities than those who simply say how the pain actually feels.

PAIN AND MEDICATION

Your pain may have a partner that shares the center of your existence: pain medication. You take your medication. It wears off. The pain returns. You take more medication. But the painkillers do more than decrease your pain; they also can improve your mood by blocking out the feelings you don't like to have. Studies have shown that with some pain medications, the effect on your mood is greater than the effect on your pain. When your pain feels worse, it is sometimes because you're upset, perhaps with your spouse or a close friend. You decide to increase your medication or take it sooner than you're supposed to. Sound familiar? If you've been there, you know what I'm talking about. If you haven't, please be aware of the pain/drug trap. It is especially dangerous when pain has replaced all the activities and relationships that made you love life. If you're taking pain medications or are thinking about it, Chapter 16 will help you understand how the various medications work.

I am not against medication to relieve pain. But pain medication is successful only if it increases your ability to function. If taking your pain pill is the highlight of your day, you're in trouble. If all the pill does is decrease your pain and does not contribute to making your life meaningful again, it isn't doing its proper job. Pain reduction without improved function is a ride to nowhere.

CHAPTER 8

Overcoming Stress and Tension

Now let's look at the list you wrote down at the beginning of the previous chapter. If you used words such as *aching, throbbing,* and *burning* (or similar words) and related the feelings to some problem in your body, you described the physical sensation of your pain. Many of you will have written phrases about your suffering and little about the actual sensation. Although we may not be able to avoid painful sensations when there is some damage in our bodies, suffering is a choice. We hope to eliminate your pain, but until that happens, let's try to minimize the suffering. Living with chronic pain does not make you into a totally different person from who you were before it took over. The pain brings out traits in yourself that were already there. Surprisingly, this can be advantageous. I have had many patients tell me that dealing with their pain gave them self-awareness, strength, and faith that they never would have achieved otherwise.

Everyone must deal with hassles in life. We have pointed to mental stress and tension as one of the reasons that muscles cause pain. We have also talked about various reasons for mental stress. To understand it further, I'd like you to answer a questionnaire. Are any of the following issues familiar? Check **yes** or **no**.

MENTAL STRESS IN YOUR LIFE

Yes No

☐ ☐ Having too much to do and too little time in which to do it.

☐ ☐ Fighting traffic to and from work.

☐ ☐ Not being sure what is expected of a job or at home.

☐ ☐ Not getting promoted; getting promoted.

☐ ☐ Never seeming to catch up financially.

☐ ☐ Being responsible for other people.

☐ ☐ Wondering if career goals are realistic.

☐ ☐ Trying to balance job demands with family responsibilities.

☐ ☐ Not being kept informed about what one needs to know to do the job.

☐ ☐ Worrying about becoming obsolete.

It's not easy getting through each day. We all need to develop skills to prevent us from being overwhelmed by all that we're expected to do. Unfortunately, we sometimes make things worse than they are. We set unrealistic expectations for ourselves. Let's look at the list below. It's an attitude assessment and comes from my first book. Check **yes** or **no** for each statement.

ATTITUDE ASSESSMENT

Yes No

☐ ☐ I can't stand it when things don't go the way I want them to.

☐ ☐ There's a perfect way to solve every difficulty.

☐ ☐ I could never change my beliefs.

☐ ☐ If I don't offer help to everyone who has a problem, I'm not a good person.

☐ ☐ If you want to be good at what you do, your goal should be to never make a mistake.

☐ ☐ Self-discipline is easy for some people, but I have never been able to succeed at it.

☐ ☐ What I look for in all of my relationships, including work, is for people to love me.

☐ ☐ If I don't try to perform better than other people, I don't think I'm performing well at all.

☐ ☐ Bad things that happened to me when I was a child will always make my life miserable.

☐ ☐ I have to be in the mood to do something, otherwise I can't do it.

☐ ☐ I'm not comfortable when I do something unless other people support me in it.

☐ ☐ You reach a point in life when you know that there's only one right way to do things.

☐ ☐ I can't stand it when somebody breaks a promise; he/she ought to be made to pay for it.

☐ ☐ Often the best thing to do in a situation is to give up.

☐ ☐ Before you take a chance, you should have a guarantee that things will turn out right.

☐ ☐ Doctors have to help me. That's their job.

☐ ☐ In choosing friends, I want only those who do things my way.

☐ ☐ I can't stand to change my feelings; I'm stuck with them.

☐ ☐ I organize my life to protect myself against change.

☐ ☐ Worrying about things that might happen helps me prepare for problems.

☐ ☐ Before I make a decision, I have to be absolutely sure that I'm making the right one.

☐ ☐ Someone has to have the cure for my problems.

☐ ☐ If there's a possibility that something bad will happen, it probably will.

☐ ☐ I can't stand it when people don't live up to what I expect of them.

☐ ☐ Life should be fair.

If you subscribe to any of these beliefs, you are holding yourself back not only from overcoming your pain but also from achieving the most happiness and fulfillment you could achieve. Life happens. We wish things would happen a certain way, but it is the way it is. Imposing any expectations on how things will turn out is sowing the seeds of resentment and disappointment. Do not let these issues make your pain worse. You may not have the power to control your pain, but you do have the power to accept life and to make it work for you. If you have ever believed that your life had meaning, then live your life as if you still do, and you will find the way to do it. Never give up. What was your purpose before you had pain? How will you live so that you have integrity for the things you stand for?

Thomas Edison failed ten thousand times before he finally invented the light bulb. He never gave up. He never felt that any failure was evidence that he had failed in life. You can have a positive, meaningful, fulfilled, happy, and productive life in spite of your back pain, if you accept the things you can't change, change the things you can, and achieve the wisdom to know the difference.

Your struggles may be fierce. Sometimes we lose faith in ourselves, in those around us, in life, and in God if you believe in God. Sometimes we are overcome by fear. But fear is a faith of its own: the faith that nothing will ever work out. The bottom line is, if you are struggling with your life for any reason, giving in to fear will cause muscle tension, create negative perceptions and feelings, and ultimately increase your pain and your inability to function.

Something that helps when you are struggling with fear and stress is to make sure that you get enough physical activity. Studies have shown that people who exercise have less anxiety, depression, and a greater feeling of well-being—besides all the physical benefits such as weight control and lowered blood pressure—than those who don't exercise. Everyone needs enough exercise and sleep. If you have pain, you need it even more.

The twenty-one Kraus-Marcus exercises outlined in Chapter 10, along with a walking program and eight hours of sleep at night, will help improve your mood and outlook. You will feel more alive and think more clearly.

If sleep is a problem and an increase in your activity level is not enough to help you restore a healthy pattern of sleep, you should speak to your doctor about a temporary addition of the right sleep medication. Natural remedies are preferable, such as chamomile tea or warm milk if they work for you. But the bottom line is this: poor sleep will increase your stress level and is associated with increased muscle pain.

Do you remember my patient Allison? You may recall that as her pain decreased, she became sad and started to cry, and soon after, her pain returned. Well, she is now pain free.

Here is what happened: at first, when I asked her what she was thinking, her crying was slight. But when I told her there must be something in her life that has been troubling her, she began to sob.

"It's my baby brother," she said. "I am afraid he's giving up on his life." Her brother was twenty years old. "He wants to be an artist, and my parents are demanding he stay in school. He had a depression so serious he had to be hospitalized, and I don't know what is going to happen."

I asked about her childhood. She told me that as the eldest of her siblings, she felt responsible for the others when her parents were busy, which was frequent. She realized, as we spoke, that she felt responsible for everyone who was important in her life. She said that she even felt compelled to give advice to almost everyone she knew. Before her pain developed, the usual smile and customary energy she exhibited hid a constant feeling of pressure and dread that something bad would happen to someone dear to her.

Thinking about all of that, she said through her sobs, "My pain in my pelvis started when my brother was hospitalized for depression." Allison continued to cry and then told me that her pain was almost gone.

I continued to explore with Allison how her beliefs about her power to control people and their lives were not realistic. She began to see that her experiences as a child colored her life as an adult and, more important, that she could start to think differently. At the same time, we continued treatment with the last level of the exercises in Chapter 10. After four weeks, Allison returned to her usual gym routine at about 40 percent of the workout that she used to do before her back pain developed. Since then, she has slowly regained all her strength and endurance, but, happily, not her pain.

Allison's expectations and defenses were all based on the model of her relationship to her family. Being in pain and being forced to rely on others was a humiliation and defeat almost as painful as the back pain itself. Allison may never have reached this realization on her own. Her pain was a gift in disguise. Her healing insight was a direct result of the courage to face the repressed issues connected to the total pain in her life. Allison's back pain was related only partly to her strained, tense muscles. Her lifelong emotional pain had become mixed in with her physical pain. If she had not had to struggle to overcome her back pain, she might never have been able to free herself from believing that she could save everyone. Allison learned to appreciate the power of her feelings. I suggested that psychotherapy could further help her see how much her childhood had defined her beliefs.

What is your secret burden? What recurring thought or feeling associated with resentment, fear, shame, guilt, and/or disappointment do you have? Perhaps this is your chance to take the sting out of events in your past that have stayed with you. Maybe your pain will be a gift in disguise.

CHAPTER 9

Test Yourself with the Kraus-Weber Tests

The Kraus-Weber tests, which will allow you to see if you meet the minimum standard of physical fitness for daily living, were originally developed for children. In 1940, Dr. Sonja Weber observed the increasing prevalence of poor posture in children and started the Posture Clinic at Columbia-Presbyterian Medical Center in New York City. She invited Hans Kraus to join her.

Dr. Weber's father was Dr. Theodor Escherich, who had been a pediatrician at St. Anna Children's Hospital in Vienna. He was concerned about the high childhood mortality rates from intestinal diseases. In 1886, he made one of the landmark discoveries in the history of medicine when he found a critically important bacterium in children's feces, later named *Escherichia coli*, or *E coli*. As a result of this discovery, health authorities around the world began the practice of monitoring the levels of *E coli* in water supplies to guard the public against water polluted with raw sewage containing feces.

Drs. Weber and Kraus were to make their own important contribution to medical knowledge by recognizing the impact of the deteriorating state of physical fitness of "advanced" sedentary societies throughout the world. The Posture Clinic lasted four years and studied two hundred children; 10 percent had congenital problems in their spine to account for their posture, but in the remaining 90 percent, there was no obvious cause. Told to stand erect, they readily did so, but the minute Kraus and Weber turned away, they slumped. The two doctors took photographs and measurements, and then they speculated that perhaps something was wrong with the youngsters' muscles.

A battery of tests was devised—originally fifteen of them—to measure the strength and flexibility of the back, belly, and hip muscles used to hold the body erect. This took years, during which time the doctors prescribed exercises to see if posture improved. Finally, they reduced the number of test exercises to six in what is now known as the Kraus-Weber (K-W) tests, and they gave the children specific therapeutic exercises designed to correct the muscular deficiencies identified on the K-W.

The K-W tests worked to identify those whose postural muscles were weak or stiff, regardless of age, weight, height, or family background. The children who practiced the prescribed exercises developed good posture, while those who started and stopped again slumped and slouched. "Although Kraus's work with children at the Posture Clinic was gratifying, he started to wonder whether weak or tense muscles might cause other types of problems for children or adults," writes biographer Susan E. B. Schwartz in her book *Into the Unknown*. Then a more serious and widespread challenge caught his interest.

"Just at the time World War II was ending, a new epidemic was striking America for the first time. Few ever heard of it before the war. Now it struck seemingly out of the blue, hitting indiscriminately across all demographic lines. No one knew where it came from, what caused it, or how to stop it. Finding its causes, prevention, and cure would occupy the rest of Kraus's life. The epidemic was back pain."

Muscles, tendons, and ligaments are the sources of most back pain. The main problem with muscles is not a specific disease but rather a state of deconditioning. A healthy muscle will be strong and flexible. Strength without flexibility produces a muscle that can be injured and cause pain more easily. Flexibility has two major components: physiological elasticity and mechanical elasticity. Physiological elasticity is the ability of the muscle to eliminate all voluntary contraction; in other words, to completely let go. Mechanical elasticity is the ability of the muscle to stretch. The flexibility that you experience in your body is based on your ability to let go and stretch. When you are relaxed, the next part of getting loose is to limber, which is to move within the range of comfort and then actively stretch the muscle. When working with a therapist, the last bit of flexibility can be produced by gentle passive stretching. Muscle strength is the ability of the muscle to contract to overcome resistance, gravity, and weight.

If the muscles that support and move our spine are deconditioned, they may be the reason for back pain. The specific muscles that bend, straighten, and twist the spine are layered over the back of the spine, ribs, and pelvis. Some of these muscles were discussed in Chapter 4. They all work together with the muscles in the front of the body—primarily the abdominal muscles—to produce the changes in posture we require. Many muscles working together allow subtle and complicated movements of our torso. Many of the muscles move us in more than one direction. The tests that you will be taking evaluate the performance of multiple muscles as they produce the actions necessary for normal posture.

The tests are unique because they measure strength and flexibility. The tests most often failed are the floor-touch exercises, because many individuals have stiff hamstrings and calf muscles; and the sit-ups with knees bent, because abdominal muscle weakness is so common. It is unusual for most individuals to fail the back muscle extension tests, which suggests that the notion of weak back muscles as a cause of back pain is incorrect.

Core muscles, the muscles in your abdominal wall, back, and pelvis that stabilize the spine and pelvis, are thought to be important in posture and, when weak, can be a source of low back pain. When patients tell me that they were instructed to do core strengthening exercises, I always ask if they were tested for core weakness. The answer is always no. If you don't know that you have core weakness, why would you do core strengthening? Having said that, Dr. Kraus, who passed away in 1995, and I believe that Pilates, which address core muscles, are good exercises for many patients. Not everyone will want to do the same type of exercise. If you can pass the K-W tests, do all of the exercises below without discomfort, and you enjoy Pilates, then do them, but don't ignore the issues of tension and stress. The K-W tests measure minimal strength and flexibility of key postural muscles. If you don't pass all the parts, it suggests that your back pain is associated with deconditioning. The Kraus-Marcus exercise plan, created to eliminate the test failures, will generally reduce or eliminate your back pain.

The tests and exercises were given successfully to more than three hundred thousand participants in the YMCA, as well as to President John F. Kennedy. There are no tests of muscle strength and flexibility or standard exercises for postural muscle health commonly used by the medical community. Were you tested for strength and flexibility? Did you receive a specific exercise program from your doctor to correct any deconditioning? Muscles are ignored in the community standard of back pain evaluation and treatment.

Wе are ready to begin. Let's see how you score on the K-W tests below. A family member or friend needs to assist you. The six exercises test key muscle groups to reveal whether or not you have sufficient strength to handle your own body weight and the flexibility to move comfortably no matter your age.

If you have a back problem or other health problem, consult with your doctor before you take the K-W tests. The tests are not that demanding, but checking with your physician is the wise thing to do.

The first thing you should do before taking the tests is to take it easy. Take off your shoes, make yourself comfortable, lie down on the floor or another firm surface, and relax. *Relax.* Take a few deep breaths and put your mind and body at ease. Start when you feel ready, and when you do, don't rush and don't push.

TEST 1

This test is designed to show whether the hip flexors (the muscles that bring your knee toward your chest) and lower abdominals are strong enough. You lie flat on your back with your hands clasped behind your neck and with your legs extended and touching. Keeping your knees straight, raise both feet so that your heels are ten inches above the floor, as shown here. If you can hold this position for ten seconds, you pass this test.

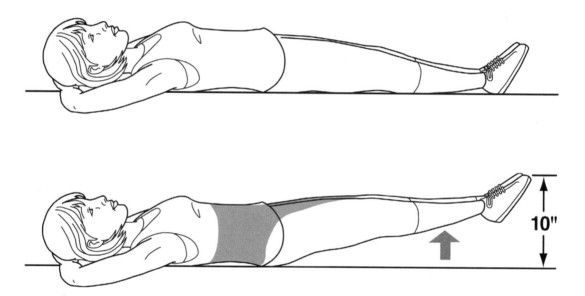

TEST 2

This test shows whether the hip flexors *and* abdominal muscles combined have sufficient strength to handle your body weight. Again lie flat with your hands clasped behind your neck. Have an assistant hold down your legs by grasping the ankles, or you can anchor your feet with heavy furniture, as shown. If you can do one sit-up by rolling up into a sitting position, you pass this test.

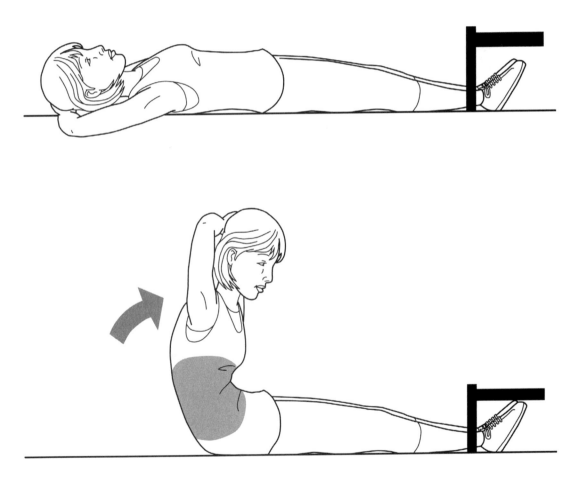

TEST 3

This tests the strength of just the abdominal muscles. As before, lie flat on the floor with your hands clasped behind your neck, only this time have your knees flexed, as shown. Have your helper hold down your ankles or anchor your feet with heavy furniture as shown. You pass if you can roll up into a sitting position.

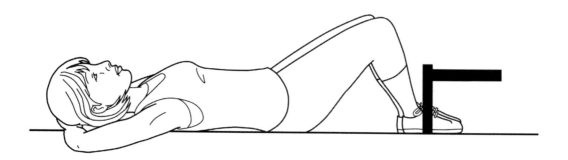

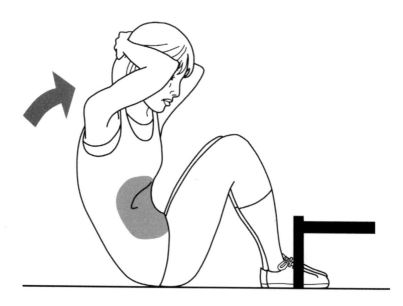

TEST 4

This tests the strength of the upper back muscles. Turn over onto your stomach.
Place a large pillow under your abdomen and hips and clasp your hands behind
your neck. Have your assistant steady the lower half of your body by placing one
hand on the small of your back and the other on your ankles. You pass if you can
lift your trunk off the floor and hold it steady for ten seconds.

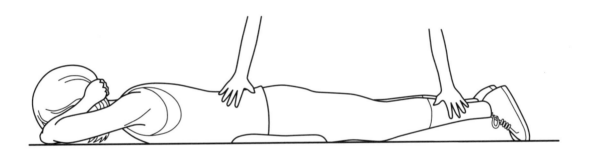

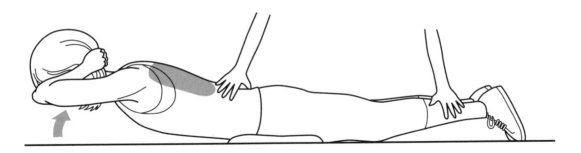

TEST 5

This tests the strength of the low back muscles. Stay on your stomach and fold your arms under your head, with the pillow still beneath your abdomen and hips. Have your assistant steady your back with both hands. You pass if you can raise your legs with the knees straight, as shown, and hold the position for ten seconds.

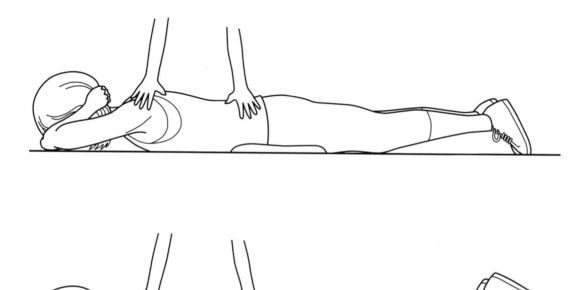

TEST 6

This tests the flexibility of the back muscles and hamstrings. Stand up straight, feet together. Slowly reach down as far as you can without bending the knees. You pass if you can touch the floor. When you come up, bend your knees so that when you raise your body, you're using your leg muscles rather than just your back muscles. If you fail, it is not because your arms are too short or your legs are too long but because the back and hamstring muscles are tense.

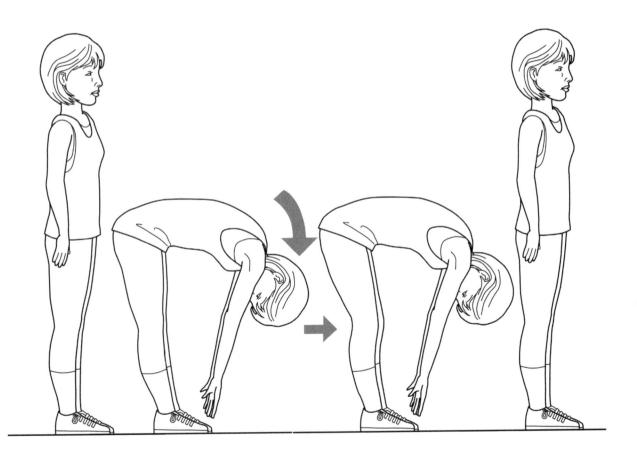

If you successfully completed all six K-W tests, you pass. You have at least met the *minimum* level of muscular fitness. If you failed even one of the six, you are below par. You are under-exercised or tense—possibly both—and you need to participate in an exercise program that can correct your deficiencies and help eliminate your pain.

CHAPTER 10

The Twenty-one Kraus-Marcus Exercises for Low Back Pain

The time has come to end your low back pain and prevent its return by starting your daily exercise program. I have modified two of the twenty-one exercises designed and developed by my mentor, Dr. Hans Kraus. They are the third and fifth exercises in level 1. I added a movement that I realized would produce a total release of the muscles controlling the thigh. It is the "frog-leg movement," and it will help you relax the adductor muscles that bring your thigh inward to the midline of your body.

The exercises are very simple. But don't let that lead you to think that they are too simple, or "sissy stuff." Forget about any other exercises that you may have done, whether it was isometrics, Pilates, jumping jacks, yoga, or pumping iron.

These exercises are specifically for you because they are *therapeutic* exercises. They are designed to correct any deficiencies revealed by the Kraus-Weber tests, regardless of whether your muscles are weak, tense, or stiff, in your back, hips, legs, or stomach.

Although these are simple exercises, consult with your doctor to ensure that you do not have a medical condition that could make them inappropriate for you.

Tens of thousands of people with low back pain have successfully performed these daily exercises. One of them was Hans's patient President John F. Kennedy. Starting at age twenty-seven, Kennedy had two disastrous spine surgeries to treat his long-standing back pain before he entered the Oval Office. Hans was called in by White House physicians Admiral George Burkley and endocrinologist Eugene Cohen, MD, who regarded Hans as "one of the great unsung medical pioneers of the century." At the time, Kennedy's back pain was so debilitating that Secret Service agents thought that he would end up in a wheelchair.

On Hans's first visit to the White House, in October 1961, he found that Kennedy's back muscles were getting stiffer and weaker, that his leg muscles were "as taut as piano wires," and that his abdominal muscles had atrophied to such a degree that he could not do even a single sit-up. As an added complication, Hans learned that the president was secretly being treated for Addison's disease, which is caused by adrenal gland failure and at that time was frequently fatal. To offset the disease, Kennedy was receiving cortisone injections that gave him a tanned, puffy face.

Hans told Kennedy that he would need to visit the White House three days a week in order to treat his back pain successfully. The president balked. He had denied to the press that he had Addison's disease and kept the crutches he used for his back hidden. He was concerned that regular visits by Hans would prompt reporters to write that the president actually had health problems.

"It's your decision," Hans replied. "But when you get worse, what will they write then?" Kennedy not only relented, he had a red telephone installed in Hans's Manhattan office in case of emergency.

Within a month after starting the exercises, Kennedy could almost touch his toes. By diligently doing the exercises, his flexibility and strength improved, his pain decreased, and for the first time Kennedy was able to pick up and toss his two-year-old son, John, in the air. Although Hans made eighty-five trips in all to the White House, he never talked to the press or asked for a fee.

Hans was, as I've said, a renowned mountaineer and rock climber in his native Austria and later in the United States. He had tried to join the Tenth Mountain Division of the US Army during World War II. He knew the Alps and the Dolomites firsthand. He was a skier. He spoke German, Italian, and French—and he was a surgeon. But even though he had fled from Austria in 1938 after the Nazi takeover, the US State Department labeled him a German enemy alien, and the army rejected him. Twenty years later, Hans felt that by treating the president he could at last repay his adopted country.

From 1976 to 1988, more than 300,000 people with low back pain—in the United States, Canada, Australia, and Japan—took part in "The Y's Way to a Healthy Back" program, based on eighteen of the twenty-one exercises that you are about to take. The largest program of its kind ever in the world, it was the brainchild of YMCA physical educator Alexander Melleby, who succeeded in getting the help and support of an originally skeptical Hans. Hans didn't think the YMCA would have the commitment to teach an exercise program on a large scale. Together they traveled across America teaching the exercises and the therapeutic rationale behind them to an initial cadre of 300 physical educators assigned to lead the six-week course.

The most detailed study of the effectiveness of the program involved 11,809 participants. After six weeks, 9,532 of them, or 81 percent, reported no pain or reduced pain. Among the 11,809 was a subset of 546 participants who had pain following surgery when they began the program. After six weeks, 83 percent reported less pain. Unfortunately, despite the great success of the program, after Melleby retired, YMCA officials allowed it to end.

The exercises are very simple, but I have found that to eliminate your low back pain, you must do them as described. First of all, set aside a time during the day when you will not be disturbed. No TV, no music, no phone calls, no conversations, no interruptions, no distractions, and no worries of any kind. This is the time for your mind and your body to relax and remain relaxed while you perform the exercises in order. You will need about ten minutes to do the first seven level 1 exercises, and then, when you add the fourteen level 2 and level 3 exercises, you will need about a half hour for the full program.

Make that your *sacred* half hour: your physical well-being and your peace of mind jointly depend upon this dedicated half hour. Don't begrudge the time; it can be your lifesaver. I have found that those patients who do best are the ones who do the exercises daily and do not skip a day. Each exercise was thoughtfully placed in the order you find it, so dropping an exercise because it seems too simple, or because you want to substitute one that you saw on TV or a friend told you about is a bad idea. These are the twenty-one exercises that you need to end low back pain, and you need to do them every day once you start. Should you run into a troubling day, a day filled with irritations, interruptions, or bad news that leaves you wired with tension, that is the very kind of day you need most to shed muscle tension and put your mind at peace.

Be as comfortable as possible. Take off your shoes and wear loose clothing that allows free movement. Lie down on your back on a firm surface. Do not use a soft mattress or a hard floor; you can hurt yourself. I recommend an exercise mat that you can place on the floor.

Regardless of how many of the exercises you do, you must always finish by repeating the exercises in reverse order. For example, every day of the first week, you are to do exercises 1 through 7, then do exercise 6 back down to exercise 1. And after you proceed from exercise 1 to exercise 21, go in reverse order from exercise 20 back down to exercise 1. *Always* complete your daily program by doing the exercises in reverse order so that your muscles are as relaxed at the finish as they were at the start.

Remember, these are *therapeutic* exercises. For them to work, you must do them smoothly. Do not strain. Be relaxed. Rid yourself of all care. As you lie down to start your daily program, think only of the exercise that you are about to do. Nothing else counts but the exercise. Do not rush. You will add the instruction "Now let go" at the end of each movement. "Letting go" means releasing all muscle tension and allowing yourself to feel like a rag doll. Let three seconds pass before repeating an individual exercise. You are not in a race. If you rush, you negate the beneficial effects. Remember: *three seconds.* This will keep you in a relaxed state of muscle and mind.

For the first week, do the level 1 exercises, 1 through 7 and back down to exercise 1. These seven exercises are designed to teach you relaxation and limbering (movement through a range of comfort). After the first week, add exercises in the order given from levels 2 and 3. By the end of the third week, most people are doing all twenty-one exercises. All exercises on your back are done in the basic position, with your knees bent, your feet flat on the mat, and your arms by your side.

LEVEL 1

RELAXATION EXERCISES

1. DIAPHRAGMATIC DEEP BREATHING

The first exercise is to help you relax through proper breathing. Lie down in the basic position: on your back, knees bent, feet flat on the mat, and your arms at your sides. Breathe in through your nose so that your stomach expands and your chest does not move. Exhale slowly through your mouth as your stomach flattens. Do this exercise three times, and be sure to wait three seconds after exhaling.

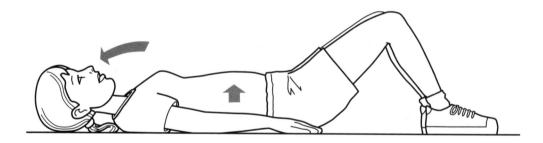

2. DEEP BREATHING WITH SHOULDER SHRUGS

This time as you breathe in through your nose, shrug your shoulders up toward your ears as far as they can go and hold for a moment. Now, as you exhale slowly through your mouth, let your shoulders return to a relaxed position. Do this three times, pausing three seconds before each successive shrug.

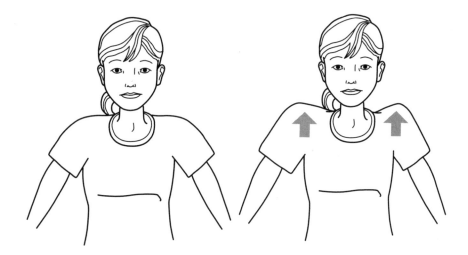

3. FROG-LEG RELEASE

On your back in the basic position, take a deep breath and exhale as you let your right leg flop to the side like the leg on a frog. Now slowly bring your right foot forward so that your right knee is pulled back toward the center. When your leg is fully extended, slowly slide it back to the basic position. Do this two more times and then do the same with the left leg three times.

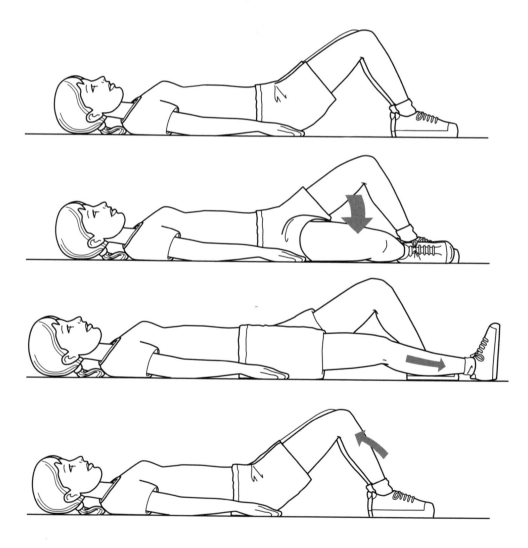

4. HEAD ROTATION

The purpose of this exercise is to relax your neck muscles. On your back in the basic position, inhale through your nose as you drop your head to the left side. When your head is all the way to the side, slowly return it to the central position, while exhaling. Now do the same as you rotate your head to the right side. Do this three times, alternating sides.

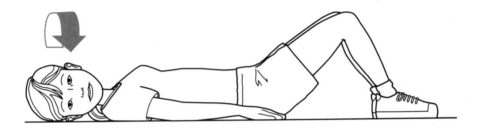

5. KNEE-TO-CHEST LEG RELEASE

This exercise is similar to the frog-leg exercise except that it has a knee-to-chest movement before the frog-leg release. On your back in the basic position, inhale as you raise your right knee as far as it can go back toward your chest. Try to keep your chest relaxed as you're doing this. Do not touch your knee with your hands. Your knee should move up on its own without any help. When it is as far back as it can go toward your chest, exhale slowly as your leg returns to the bent position. Now let your right knee flop to the side like the leg on a frog. Slide your foot down so that your leg straightens. Slide your foot back so that your leg is in the bent-knee position. Do this two more times with the right leg and then three times with the left leg.

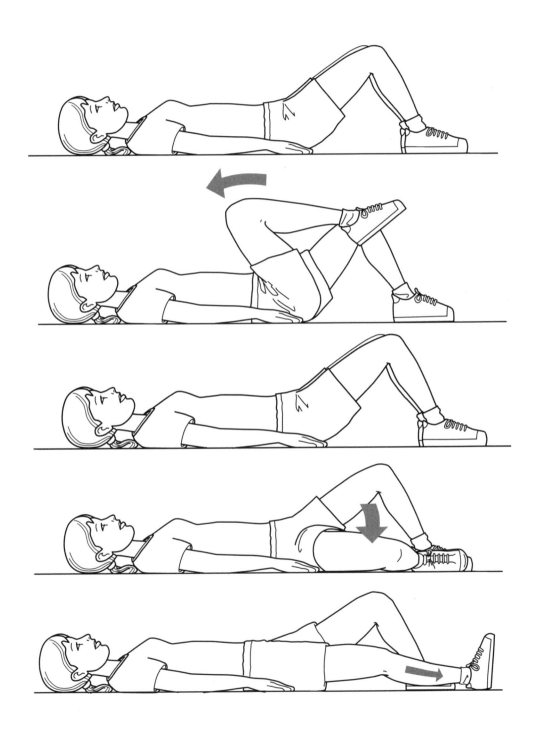

6. SIDE SLIDE

The side slide exercise is intended to limber your hip flexors and the muscles that extend and flex your legs. Lie on your left side in a relaxed semi-fetal position, with your knees bent but your upper body straight. Keep your upper body straight as you slide your right leg on your left leg up toward your chest. As your right knee passes the lower left knee, let the right knee touch the mat as you continue to slide the right knee toward your chest. *Slide* the leg; do not lift it. When your right knee has reached maximum movement toward your chest, begin to extend your right leg downward in the opposite direction. When your right leg is completely extended, slide it back to the bent position—the right knee resting on the left knee—and let go of all muscle effort for a moment. Do this exercise two more times with the right leg, then turn onto your right side and do the exercise three times with the left leg. Again, this is a *sliding* exercise. Do not lift the moving leg—and don't forget to breathe.

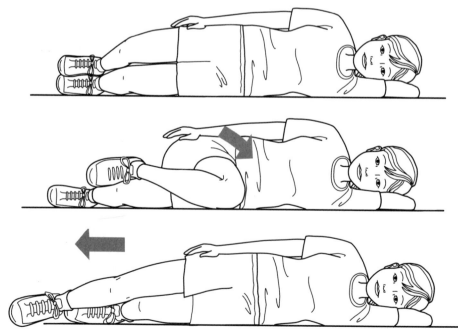

7. BUTTOCKS SQUEEZE

Lie on your stomach with a pillow underneath your pelvis to support your hips. Breathe in through your nose and squeeze your buttocks for three seconds; then exhale and let go. Do the buttocks squeeze two more times. If you have a problem feeling a tight squeeze, rotate your feet so that the toes are facing outward. As you do so, you will feel more tension in your thighs and buttocks, and when you attempt to squeeze again, you will get a tighter squeeze.

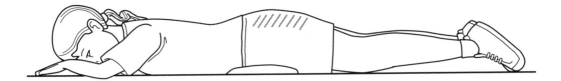

After performing the Buttocks Squeeze, complete level 1 by doing the exercises in reverse order, starting with the Side Slide.

LEVEL 2

LOWER BODY EXERCISES

After doing level 1 exercises for one week with no discomfort, start on level 2 exercises in the numbered order. Most people will have no problem with adding all seven exercises in level 2 to the seven in level 1. If you encounter discomfort while doing one of the exercises, do only the exercises up to the uncomfortable one and then do the preceding exercises in reverse order. Do this for three days before attempting to add the uncomfortable exercise. If that exercise is still uncomfortable, skip it and go on to the rest of the exercises in level 2. After doing all the exercises in level 2, try the problem exercise again. If it is still painful, skip it and go on to add level 3 exercises, avoiding any that cause you persistent discomfort. If, after doing all of levels 2 and 3 for a week, you still cannot add the uncomfortable exercise, it may be an exercise that you will not be able to do for a while. Most people can do all twenty-one exercises, but a few have to eliminate one or two of them. Now let's get started.

8. DOUBLE KNEE TO CHEST

Lie on your back in the basic position. Inhale. As you exhale, bring both knees toward your chest as far as they will go. Do not grab your legs for assistance. Slowly lower your feet back to the basic position. Do this two more times.

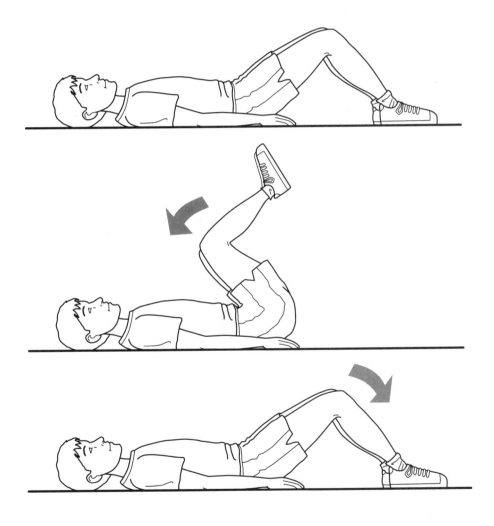

9. CAT BACK-CAMEL BACK

Turn over on your hands and knees so that they form pillars supporting your torso. Look at the illustration to see what your position should look like. Almost all the motion is done from your hips, although your spine is also involved. When you do this exercise, your legs and arms should remain vertically straight. Arch your back like a cat and let your head drop at the same time. Now lift your head and form a "U"—this is the camel back—with your spine. This exercise may be a little difficult in the beginning, particularly if you are not used to moving your hips. Don't worry about doing it perfectly. We are always more concerned with progress than perfection. If you continue to do this regularly, I promise that you'll continue to improve. So keep trying.

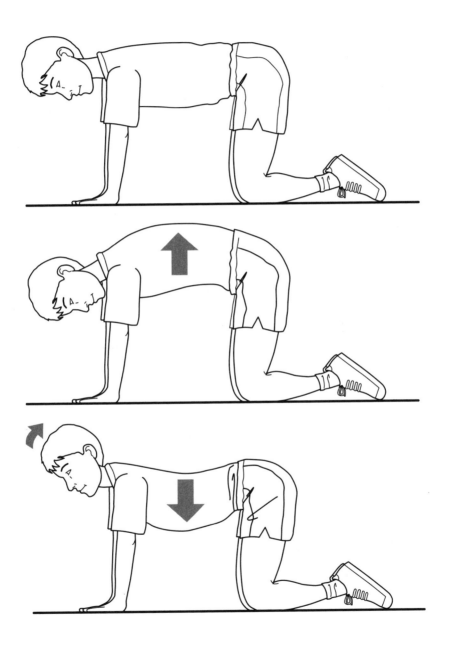

10. PARTIAL SIT-UP

Turn onto your back in the basic position. Allow your hands to rest comfortably on your thighs. Take a deep breath. As you exhale, slowly raise your head and shoulders off the mat and allow your hands to slide toward your knees. Then as you breathe in again, slowly lower your back to the basic position. One of the elements of this exercise is the breathing; when you inhale, your belly expands; and when you exhale, your belly gets sucked in, contracting the abdominal muscles. This strengthens your abdominals as you do the partial sit-up. Do the exercise two more times.

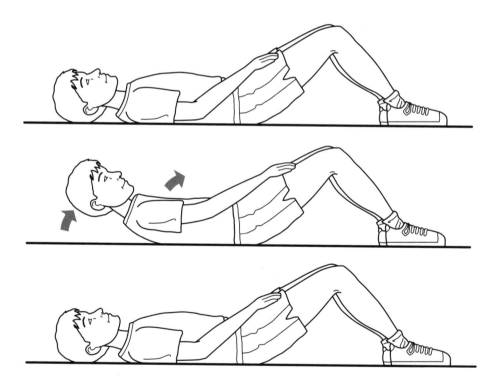

11. PECTORAL STRETCH

Study the illustration before you read the instructions for this exercise. Note that you start in a kneeling position, with your buttocks angled back toward your heels. Slide your hands forward as far as you can while keeping your head in line with your arms. In doing this pectoral stretch, you should feel a stretching sensation across the front of your chest. If you do not feel that sensation, you are not doing the exercise correctly—so repeat the exercise until you feel the stretching sensation. After you do, slowly lift your buttocks to ease the stretching sensation in your chest and repeat the process two more times. If you have shoulder or neck problems and you experience too much discomfort, eliminate this exercise.

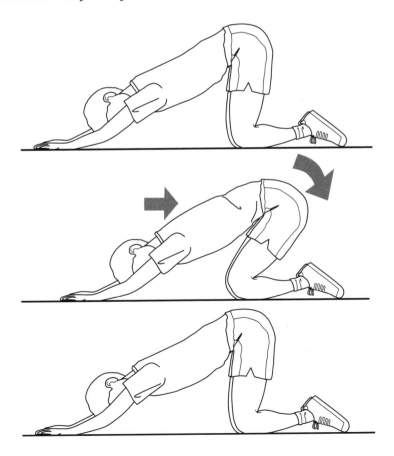

12. SEATED FORWARD BEND

This is the first exercise that you do off the mat. Find a comfortable but sturdy chair that allows you to sit with your knees bent and apart, your feet flat on the floor. Sit upright. Breathe in and out slowly several times to get relaxed. Now breathe in again. As you exhale, let your head bend forward gently to lead your trunk down toward the floor with your arms dangling in front of you between your legs as far as you can go. If your fingers cannot touch the floor, go as far down as you can without straining and then slowly roll back to the upright sitting position. Do two more times.

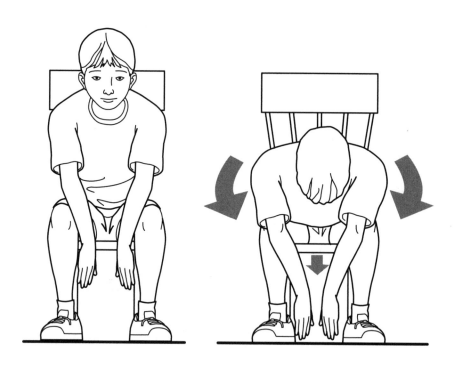

13. BICYCLE HAMSTRING STRETCH

At first, you will not be able to raise your straightened leg completely as in the figures on the next pages. With time, you will be able to slowly increase the amount you can raise your straightened leg. There are two bicycle stretch exercises. The only difference between them is the position of the foot, which determines whether the exercise focuses primarily on the hamstring or calf muscles. This first bicycle stretch focuses more on the hamstring muscles than on the calf muscles. Start on your back in the basic position. Bring your right knee to your chest as far as you comfortably can. Now straighten your leg upward, and as soon as it is entirely straight, lock your knee, with your toes pointed straight toward the ceiling. Slowly lower your straight leg to the mat. Relax and let go. Bend your knee as you slide the leg back to the basic position. Do two more times with the right leg and three times with the left leg.

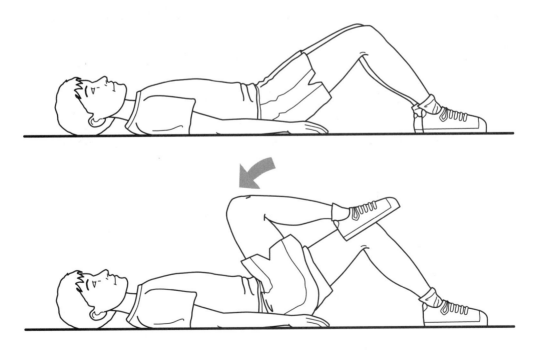

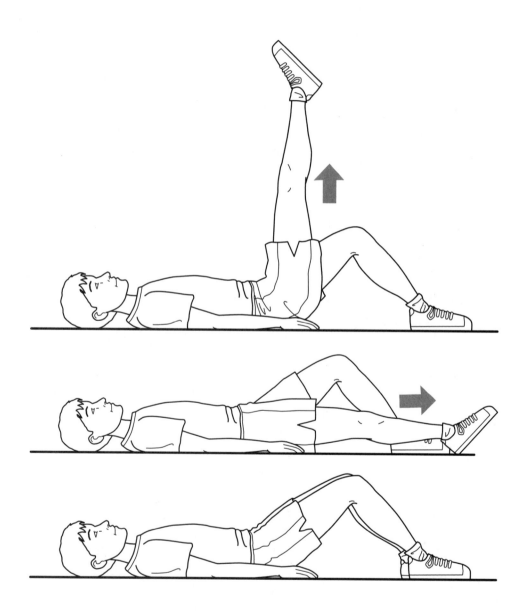

14. BICYCLE CALF STRETCH

This bicycle stretch focuses more on the calf muscles than the hamstring muscles. Starting in the basic position, bring your right knee to your chest as far as you comfortably can. Now straighten that same leg, knee locked, but this time with the ankle flexed so that the heel, not the toes, points toward the ceiling. Maintain the heel position as you slowly lower your straight leg until the heel touches the mat. Slide the heel back until the knee is bent and the foot flat on the mat in the basic position. Relax and let go. Do this twice more with the right leg and three times with the left leg.

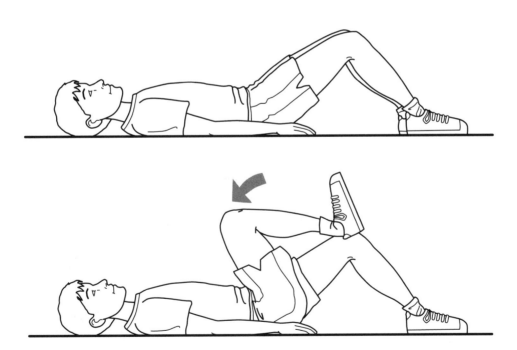

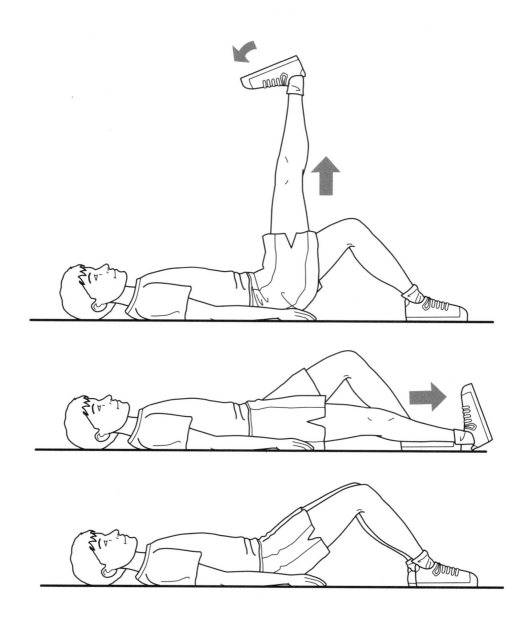

LEVEL 3

MORE S-T-R-E-T-C-H-I-N-G

The next seven exercises provide greater stretching to your trunk, hip, and leg muscles. They therapeutically follow the level 1 and level 2 exercises and should always be done after them, never before or out of sequence. Remember that twenty-one exercises constitute *the* program and are not to be done piecemeal. As I said at the beginning of this chapter, I have found that as some patients get better at doing the exercises, they tend to rush, to do "their own thing," and thus they forget or ignore the most important element in these exercises, which is relaxing and letting go. Mastering the art of relaxing and letting go can be especially difficult if you are always out to "win" in life and get what you want. To paraphrase Bob Dylan, "You may know what you want, but as a physician I know what you need."

If you are physically active, you may find the level 3 exercises more appealing because they are more difficult than the previous exercises, but let me remind you again, you must relax and let go. By doing the exercises properly, you will find them a godsend in helping you to overcome back pain and the stresses of daily living.

15. FULL SIT-UP

Begin in the basic position. You will need to anchor your feet and ankles under a sturdy chair or couch or have someone hold them down. Place your hands on either side of your face or behind your neck. If you have difficulties doing this because of neck or shoulder discomfort, put your hands on your chest. Inhale first, and as you exhale, roll your torso up toward your knees. Do this slowly and smoothly without jerking your head and shoulders to initiate the movement. Do not strain. If you are deconditioned and have never done a sit-up, do not be concerned, just do what you can. Remember, if you keep doing it, you will get better at it, and your abdominal muscles will get stronger. As you breathe in, your stomach should expand, and as you exhale, your abdominal muscles should tighten and strengthen. Then slowly roll your torso back toward the mat until you're lying with your head on the mat once again in the basic position.

If you cannot do this exercise at all, start with your arms at your sides to give you some support when you first raise your head and shoulders. You may have to do this for a few days—possibly for weeks—before your abdominals are strong enough for you to start to do a full sit-up. As you begin to develop some strength in your abs, you may place your hands on your stomach, and then as your abs get stronger, move your hands higher on your body: first on your chest and, finally, up to your face or behind your neck.

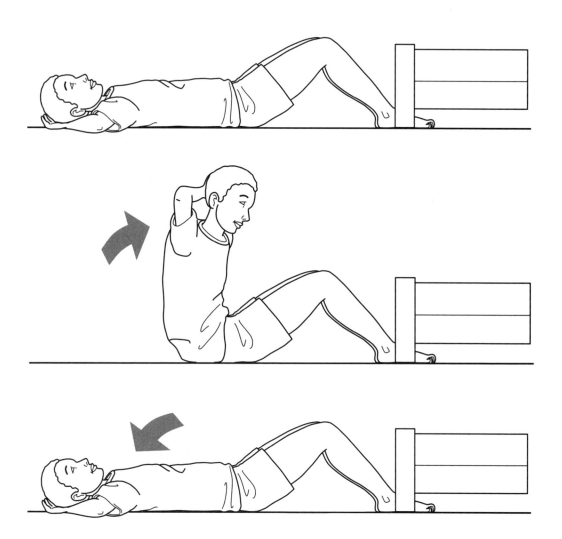

16. SEATED SIDE BEND

Start by sitting upright in a chair. Breathe in and exhale to get yourself relaxed. Now breathe in again, and as you exhale, let your head bend forward gently to lead your body down, your hands coming together on the outside of your left knee. Slide your arms downward to the left until your fingers are as close as they can come to the floor. Be careful to maintain your balance and not fall off the chair. Return to the upright sitting position, inhaling while you do so. Do this two more times to the side of your left knee and three times to the side of your right knee.

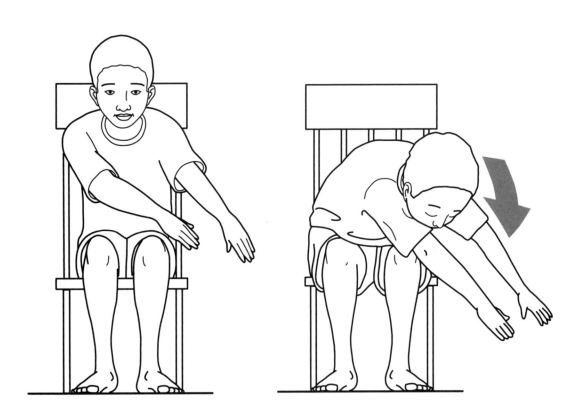

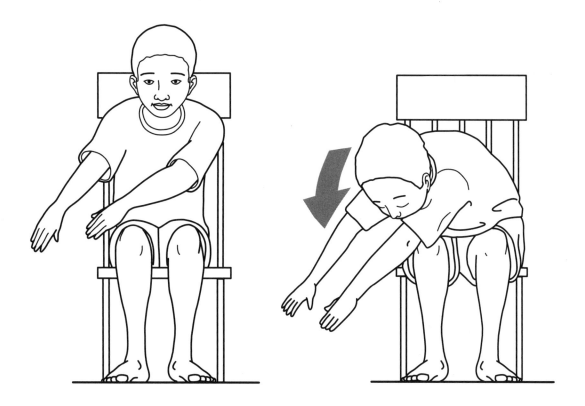

17. STRAIGHT LEG RAISE HAMSTRING STRETCH

This exercise and the one that follows are similar to the bicycle exercises, but they are more difficult because they do not have the bicycle motion to modulate the stretch. Begin in the basic position and breathe in as you slide your right leg all the way down. With your leg straight and your knee locked, exhale slowly and raise the leg as high as you comfortably can, with your foot pointed down. (Imagine walking on your toes.) Lower the straight leg. When your heel touches the mat, slide the leg back to the basic position and let go. Do this three times with each leg.

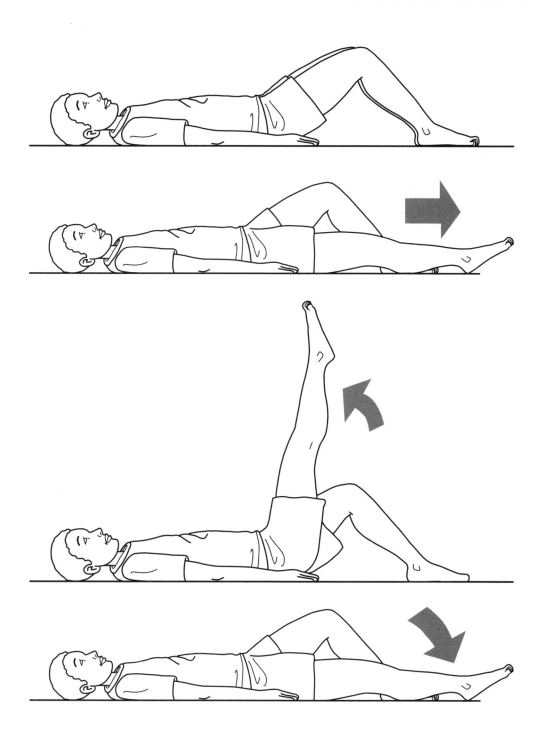

18. STRAIGHT LEG RAISE CALF STRETCH

Begin in the basic position and breathe in as you slide your right leg all the way down, with your foot and toes pointed up. (Imagine walking on your heel.) With your leg straight and your knee locked, exhale slowly as you raise the leg as high as you comfortably can, with the foot still pointed up. Lower the straight leg, and when the heel touches the mat, slide the leg back to the basic position and let go. Do this three times with each leg.

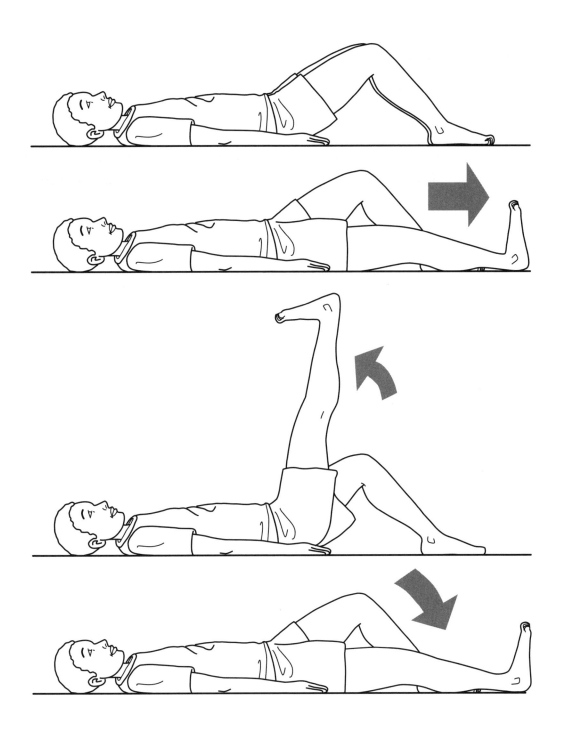

19. DIVER'S BEND

Stand up, with your feet slightly apart. Clasp your hands behind your back. Bend forward from the hips, keeping your back, neck, and knees straight. Bend as far as you can and then raise your head until you feel a stretching sensation in the back of your legs. Now raise your arms off your back and move them up toward the ceiling to increase the stretching sensation in your calves. Then bend your knees slightly and slowly roll up to the upright position.

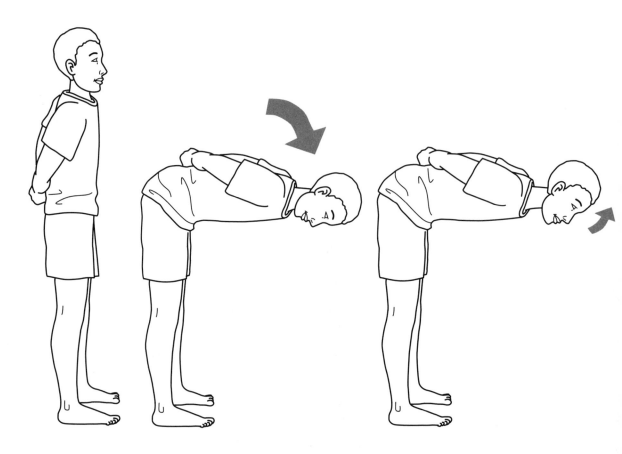

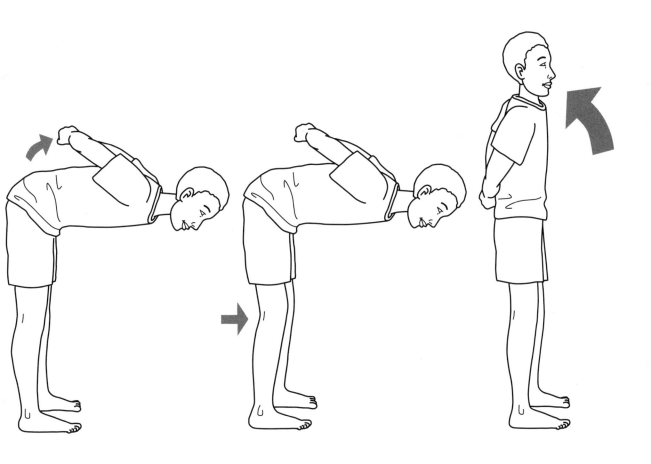

20. WALL CALF STRETCH

Stand facing a wall, approximately eight to ten inches away. Place your palms on the wall with your arms fully extended. Take a deep breath, bend your elbows, and exhale, while keeping your back and hips straight and your feet parallel and flat on the floor. You should feel the stretch in your calf muscles when you do this. If you do not feel the stretch in your calf muscles, you are not far enough away from the wall, so move back a few inches until you begin to feel the stretch in the calves. Now that you're the correct distance from the wall, bend your elbows again and go as far as you can toward the wall, making sure that you do not lose your balance. Your back and hips should be straight; your feet should be parallel and flat on the floor. Make sure that your heels are firmly touching the floor. Once you've gone as far as you can, straighten your arms to push your body back to an erect standing position. The stretch portion of the exercise—when you're in the process of bending your elbows—is done while exhaling.

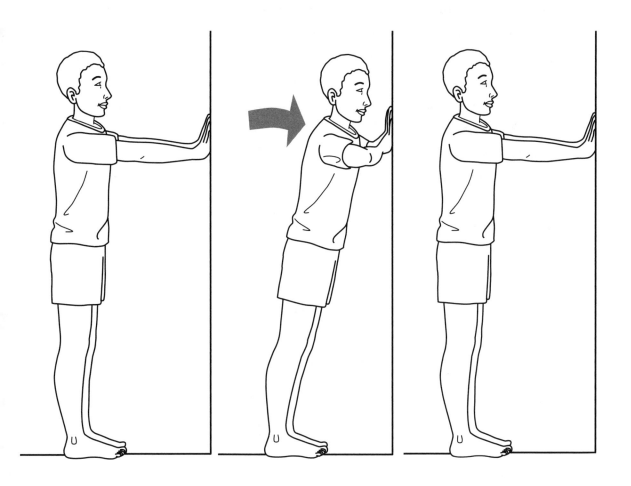

21. FLOOR TOUCH

*S*tand with your feet together and legs straight. Inhale, and as you slowly exhale, let your head droop. Bend down as far as you can, with your knees locked and feet together. Try to touch the floor with your outstretched fingertips without bouncing or forcing yourself. (Your fingertips may be more than a foot from the floor when you first start doing this exercise.) Once you are as far down as you can go, bend your knees and slowly roll yourself back up to the upright position. If you have great difficulty in bending over with your feet close together, spread your feet apart as much as you need to allow more downward motion. As you become more flexible, gradually move your feet closer to each other until they are finally together when you can touch the floor.

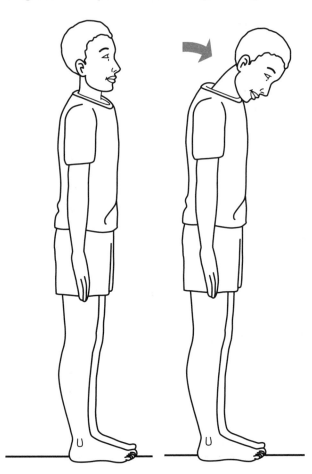

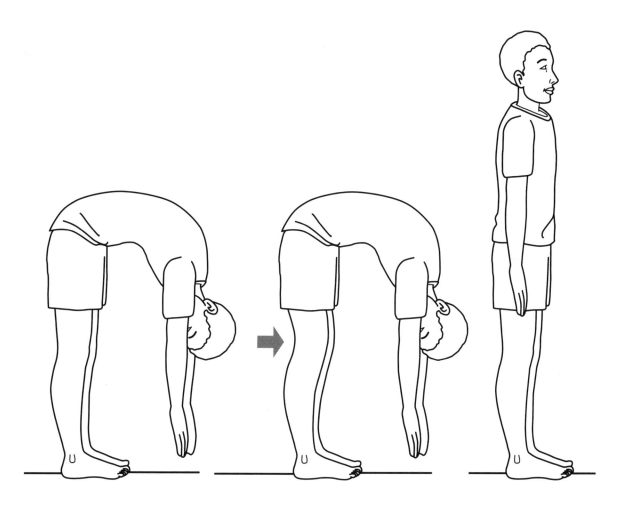

CHAPTER 11

Upper Body Exercises for Upper Back, Shoulder, and Neck Pain, and Tension Headaches

The knee bone connected to the thigh bone . . .
The shoulder bone connected to the back bone . . .
—"Dem Dry Bones," Gospel song

Everything in the body is connected. To understand the whole, we need to look at the parts. Upper back pain often arises from various muscles in the upper body—some that you'd never imagine. In fact, even lower back pain can sometimes be traced to muscles above.

We can easily and simply test for muscle function in the upper body. The following tests of flexibility have helped me understand and treat my patients with upper back and body pain. The tests measure the flexibility of the neck, jaw, and shoulder, and help me identify which muscles may be contributing to your upper back and midback pain. The exercises that follow will correct many of the deficiencies that we might find doing the tests.

FORWARD FLEXION: Test one arm at a time if it is too uncomfortable raising both arms together. Fully straighten your arms. Raise them straight ahead as far as you can. Full range is 180 degrees, which would bring your arm up to the level of your ear. Compare the two sides. A difference suggests stiffness in the shoulder that could be related to your shoulder joint or to the muscles surrounding your shoulder. If there is no noise, called *crepitus*, in your shoulder as you move and no pain in the shoulder joint, chances are the stiffness is from muscles.

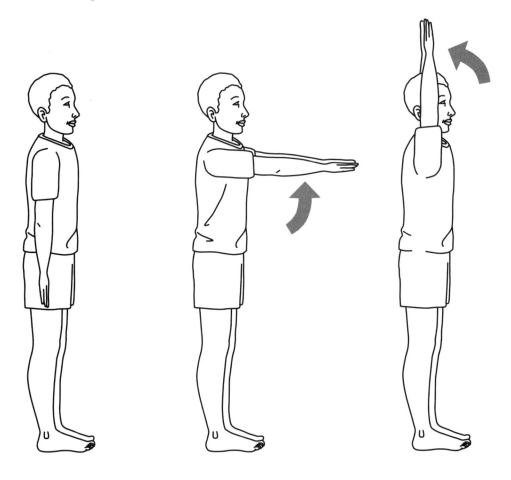

ABDUCTION: The movement of a straightened arm (or leg) away from the center of the body. Test one arm at a time if it is too uncomfortable raising both. Raise your outstretched arm sideways until it touches your ear. Going all the way is normal; less reflects a problem in your joint or muscles just as in forward flexion (as seen previously).

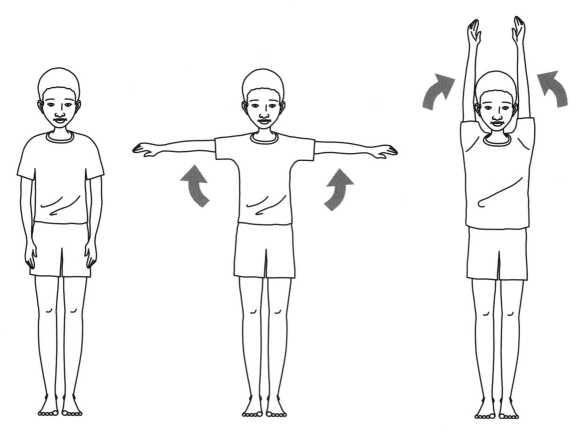

Movement of the arm and shoulder is complicated. The scapula (shoulder blade) moves on the chest, and the arm moves in the joint in the scapula. These two different shoulder movements are called: scapulo-humeral—the upper arm bone (humerus) moves in the cup of the shoulder blade, and scapulo-thoracic—the entire scapula moves on the chest (thorax). The rotation of the bone in the center of the upper arm in the shoulder joint is called internal or external rotation. You can see an illustration of the bones of the arm and shoulder in figure 23 in the insert.

INTERNAL ROTATION: Bend your elbow and reach behind you. Now, as you continue to touch your back, raise your hand up toward your neck and have a friend make a note of the highest point that you can go without using your other hand to help. Now do the other side and compare the two points. If one side is less, the distance between the two points is the deficit in functional internal rotation. The infraspinatus, teres major, rhomboids, and trapezius muscles are frequently involved in causing this deficit.

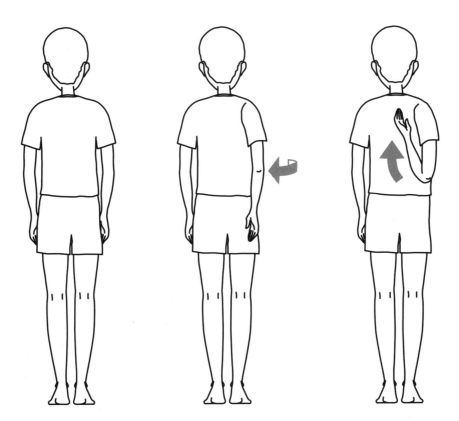

EXTERNAL ROTATION: Test one arm at a time. Bend your elbow and reach up in front of your chest to the top of your shoulder, and then down toward your lower back as far as you can go. Mark the point of greatest movement down. Do the same with the other arm. Compare the two sides. The difference is the deficit in functional external rotation of the side that moves the least. Muscles often involved in this deficit are the pectoralis major and minor, trapezius, triceps, and the latissimus dorsi. If both sides are stiff, you may not get a true picture of the apparently good side. Even though your painless side moves more than the bad side, it still may be stiff itself.

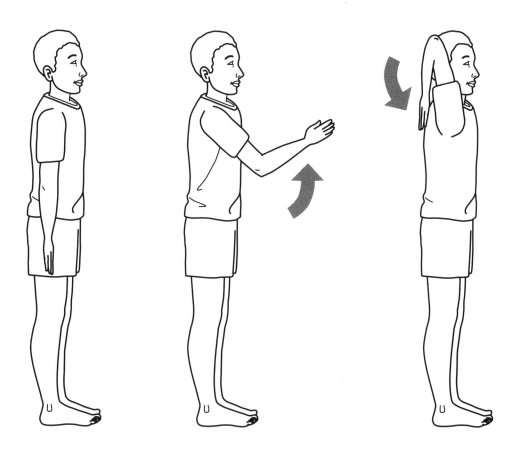

CERVICAL SPINE: Test while sitting.

1. *Flexion*: Bring your chin toward your chest. If you touch, this is full range of motion (50° is normal).

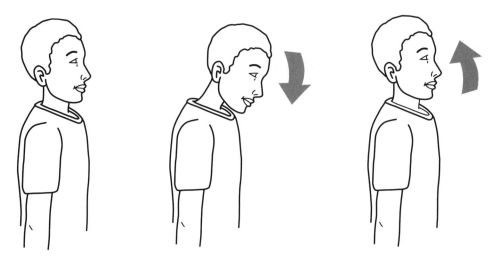

2. *Extension*: Bend your head backward toward your back (60° is normal).

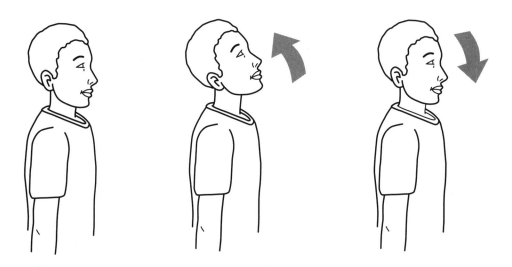

3. ***Lateral bend***: Looking straight ahead, bend your head to one side so that your ear moves directly down toward the top of your shoulder; now to the other side (45° is normal).

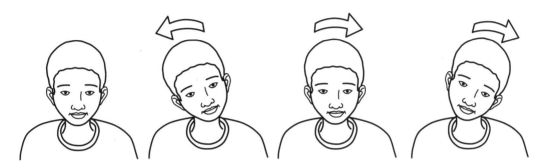

4. ***Rotation***: Keeping your eye on a line of objects in front of you at eye level, turn your head to the side as far as it will go; now to the other side (80° is normal). If you're past forty years old, you will probably feel some stiffness or pain and maybe hear a click or pop, reflecting some arthritic changes and stiff muscles in the neck. These changes come with age and for most of us, as with similar signs of aging in the lower spine, will not interfere significantly with our lives. If there is a sharp, specific pain in one spot, and it travels into an arm and down into your fingers, it may represent a nerve being squeezed in the neck. This may require attention from your doctor. Fortunately, this is usually not the case, and most of the pain and stiffness that we will encounter is from the muscles in and around the neck.

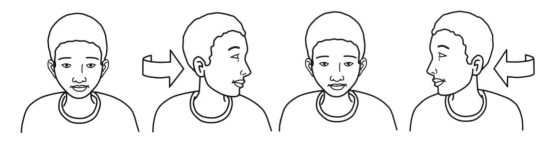

TEMPOROMANDIBULAR JOINT (TMJ): Open your mouth as wide as possible. Slowly close it and observe if the motion is a straight line or if your jaw tends to move to one side and then the other. If this is the case, the bone (mandible) in the TMJ may be moving in the socket. If there is pain at the same time, you may have a problem in the TMJ. Fortunately, most of the time, the uneven movement we observe is from muscles surrounding the joint rather than from problems in the joint. *Temporomandibular joint dysfunction* (TMD) for any reason can cause pain in your neck, shoulders, and upper back.

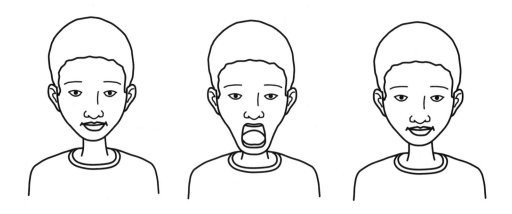

UPPER BODY EXERCISES

Before you begin these eight exercises for the upper body, be sure to review the guidelines in the previous chapter on how to make yourself as comfortable as possible. Put cares away, relax, and immerse your mind and muscles in the movements shown and described below. The exercises that follow are designed to correct muscle deficiencies that can cause pain in the upper body.

Let's start with the shoulder, where the surrounding muscles can become strained. An important part of the shoulder is the rotator cuff, which is an extension of the tendons of four muscles: infraspinatus, supraspinatus, teres minor, and subscapularis. If you follow baseball, you know that players, pitchers especially, often undergo surgery for a torn rotator cuff. In point of fact, unless the tear is major, it may not be the reason for pain and stiffness in the shoulder. What's more, therapeutic exercise for painful, stiff muscles may restore full range of motion and power to the shoulder, rendering surgery unnecessary.

Overuse and misuse of muscles in the upper body often lead to pain. Sustained contraction in a muscle—any muscle, even in a hand—is not only an invitation to pain, it can cause pain without a person being aware of the source. Here is an interesting example of how overuse can cause pain and how easy the solution may be:

A patient of mine complained of baffling pain in her left arm and shoulder. She lived in the country and routinely drove long distances to shop, and even longer distances to visit her sister on weekends. In the course of treating her, I learned that she tended to grip the steering wheel with one hand. And that, it turned out, was the problem. Her tight grip on the wheel caused the pain to radiate up her arm and into her shoulder. The solution was simple: use both hands on the steering wheel and relax the grip.

Although not as common as low back pain, chronic upper back and neck pain can come from stiff, weak, and tense muscles. Tension headaches, which affect almost 80 percent of the general population, can stem from tight muscles in the shoulder, neck, and even in your scalp and chewing muscles. These muscles that surround our jaw are the most common reason for the diagnosis temporomandibular joint dysfunction. Patients with TMD often grind their teeth at night (bruxism). If you think you may have TMD, a dentist specializing in jaw pain may be able to help you with a bite plate, a plastic appliance that protects your teeth and muscles.

There are only eight upper body exercises in my course of exercises, and they are deceptively simple. I say "deceptively" because although the movement you are asked to do looks uncomplicated, it will cause you to use muscles that you may not have used fully for years. You may be surprised to find that the stiffness prevents fluid movement in your neck and shoulders.

The importance of upper body stiffness cannot be overstated. I saw a seventy-year-old man whom I shall call Louis, who was hospitalized for twelve days for severe chest pain. His pain began in his right upper back and spread to the left side. Since he'd had a coronary-artery bypass graft (an operation to graft a new section of an artery in the heart to bypass a blocked artery, commonly called a CABG), it was feared that his pain was from his heart, even though it began on the right side. When an angiogram (an X-ray procedure that involves inserting a tube into an artery in your leg and threading it up into the arteries of your heart in order to inject a contrast dye to see if there is a blockage) showed no heart problem, he had imaging of his neck, chest, abdomen, and pelvis, visits by four specialists, and steroid injections into the painful area without any pain relief. He was given strong morphine-like medication, an anticonvulsant, and a drug for muscle spasming, all of which made him sleepy and lose his appetite, but didn't affect his pain.

When I examined Louis, I found that he could not raise his right arm while straightened so that it was at the level of his ear, but he could on the left. He could also reach behind him and up toward his neck three inches higher on his left side than his right. He had what we call frozen shoulder. He didn't know about his stiffness. The specific restrictions told me that his pain was probably coming from a muscle on top of his shoulder blade, the infraspinatus. I have found that the infraspinatus is the muscle that most often causes pain in the shoulder. I examined him with an instrument I invented, which I will share with you in Chapter 19, and found that, indeed, the infraspinatus was causing his pain. I discovered years ago that in less than two minutes, I could eliminate the pain for hours by applying a cream containing ketamine, an unusual and potent pain medication, and lidocaine, a drug that produces numbness. The cream works only for specific causes of muscle pain, most often the type of pain identified with my instrument. It worked on this patient, and he left the consultation pain free and amazed that a pain that he feared came from a not-yet diagnosed severe illness could be eliminated by treating one muscle in his shoulder.

The key to helping Louis was the physical examination, which led to the culprit muscle. The key to preventing recurrence lies in the exercises I showed him and will show you.

Before I do that, it is important to know how Louis became so stiff. I asked him if he'd had injuries to his upper body. He didn't. He'd been a truck driver for more than thirty years. Louis didn't have to lift or carry anything as part of his job. He never exercised. His job only required that he move his arms, shoulders, and neck in a limited way. This is the perfect set-up for stiffness. If we don't put our muscles through their full range of motion, they will become stiff in the areas where they never or rarely move, and you would never know about it if you weren't doing anything that would make you aware of the stiffness. If you were exercising regularly to remain flexible and strong, you would notice the areas that were not, and you could get better, as Louis will, now that he properly exercises his upper body.

Now let's go to the exercises.

All exercises should be repeated three times; four if you feel up to it.

1. DIAPHRAGMATIC DEEP BREATHING

The first exercise is intended to make you relax and breathe properly—a crucial step. Lie down in the basic position on your back, knees bent, feet flat on the mat, and your arms at your sides. Breathe in through your nose so that your stomach expands. Exhale slowly through your mouth as your stomach goes flat. Do this exercise three times, pausing three seconds before each succeeding exercise.

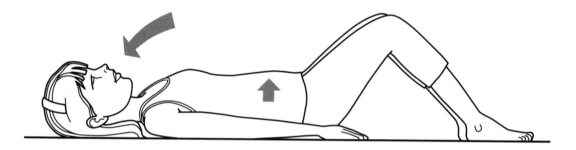

2. DEEP BREATHING WITH SHOULDER SHRUGS

This time, as you breathe in through your nose, shrug your shoulders toward your ears as far as they can go and hold for a moment. Now as you exhale slowly through your mouth, let your shoulders return to a relaxed position. Do this three times, pausing three seconds before each succeeding exercise.

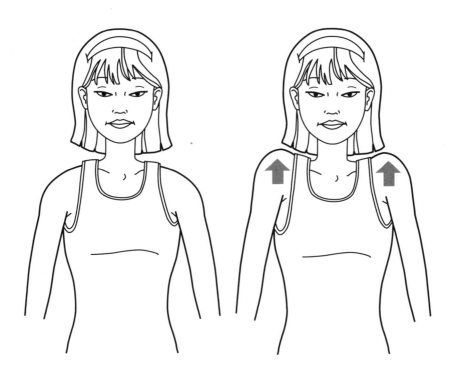

3. HEAD ROTATION

The purpose of this exercise is to relax your upper body and move your neck muscles. On your back in the basic position, inhale through your nose as you drop your head to the right side. When your head is all the way to the side, return it to the neutral position, exhaling as you do. Now do the same as you rotate your head to the left side. Do this exercise three times, alternating sides.

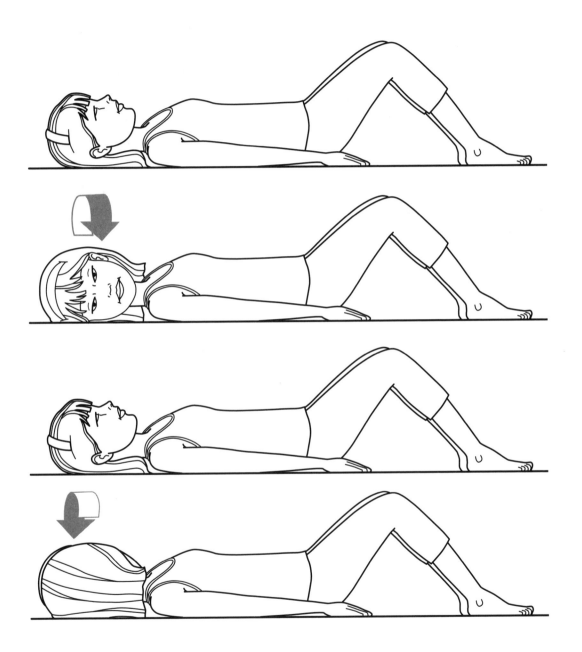

4. TENSE/RELAX

Lie on your back with your arms at your sides and your legs extended on the mat. Breathe in deeply through your nose; as you do, make two fists as tight as you can and bend your elbows, bringing your fists as close as you can to your shoulders. Now open your hands as you bring your forearms to the upright position, and then let your arms drop to the mat. Letting go of tension is the most important part of this exercise; it teaches you what it feels like to stop contracting your muscles. Focus on the sensation of letting go. Realize you can have this state of relaxation at other times. Do this exercise two more times.

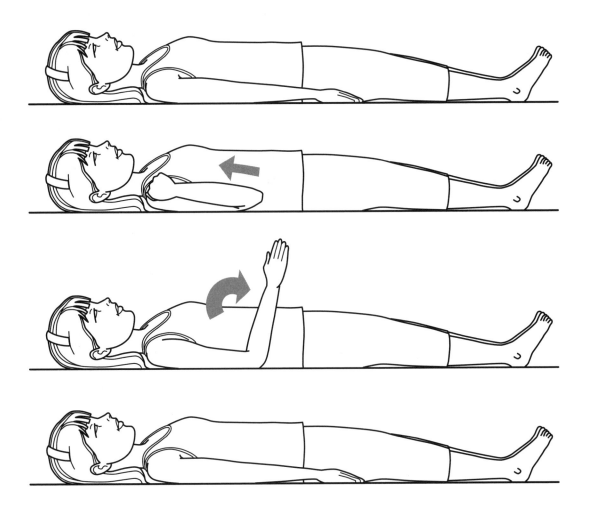

5. CHICKEN WINGS

Lie on your back with both hands on your chest and your legs extended on the mat. Breathe in deeply through your nose. Now breathe out slowly as you slide your elbows out to the sides and up as far as you can toward your ears—all the while keeping your hands on your chest. Now breathe in as you slide your elbows back to their original position. Repeat this exercise two more times.

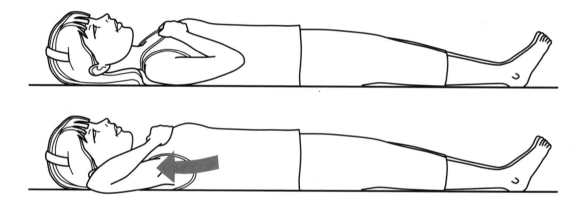

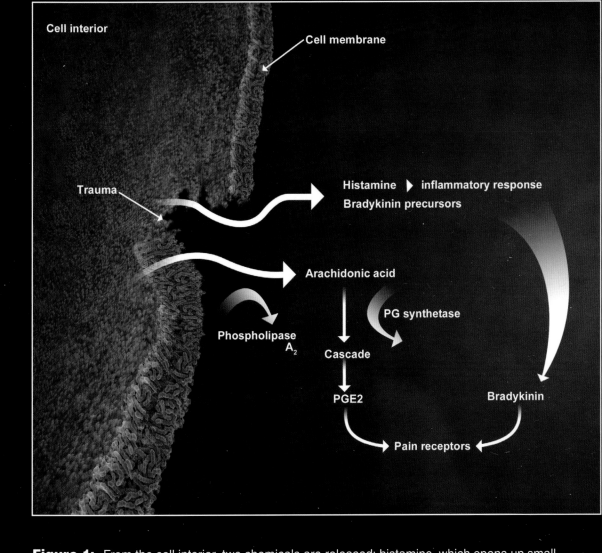

Figure 1: From the cell interior, two chemicals are released: histamine, which opens up small blood vessels and causes redness, and a chemical that will be converted to bradykinin. From the cell surface (membrane), chemicals are released that are converted into arachidonic acid, which in turn is transformed into prostaglandins (PGE2). (Over-the-counter pain drugs such as ibuprofen and naproxen work by blocking this reaction and thus blocking the production of prostaglandins.) This transformation process is called the arachidonic cascade. The prostaglandins and bradykinin together stimulate nociceptors, which transmit information to the spinal cord, telling the body that damage has occurred.

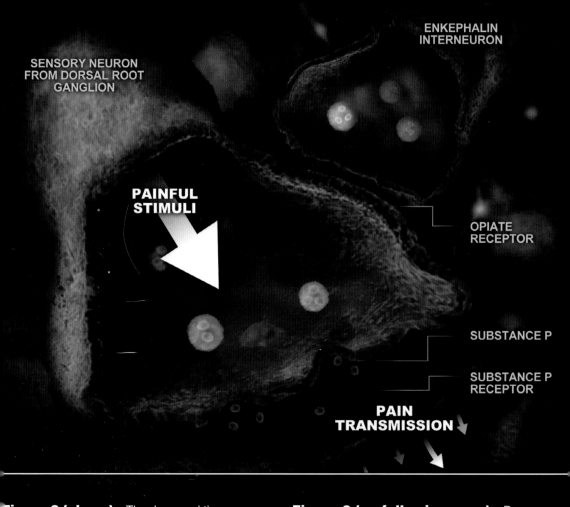

SENSORY NEURON FROM DORSAL ROOT GANGLION

ENKEPHALIN INTERNEURON

PAINFUL STIMULI

OPIATE RECEPTOR

SUBSTANCE P

SUBSTANCE P RECEPTOR

PAIN TRANSMISSION

Figure 2 (above): The damaged tissue causes a potentially painful stimulus to come into the spinal cord and release substance P (SP), which stimulates the next nerve that will send information in a path called the spinothalamic tract up to the brain. The pain mechanism is self-regulating to minimize the pain sensation so that we are not too overburdened with discomfort. You can see another nerve, which can inhibit pain transmission by releasing a morphine-like substance (enkephalins), which can block the effect of SP.

Figure 3 (on following page): Damage somewhere in your body excites pain receptors that transmit a signal to a part of the spinal cord called the dorsal horn. Substance P is released, which stimulates the next nerve in the chain on its way up to the brain. The next major station is the thalamus, the switchboard, which then transmits and receives information from the limbic system (which contributes the emotional component to your pain), and the sensory cortex (the part of the brain that tells us where the pain is located).

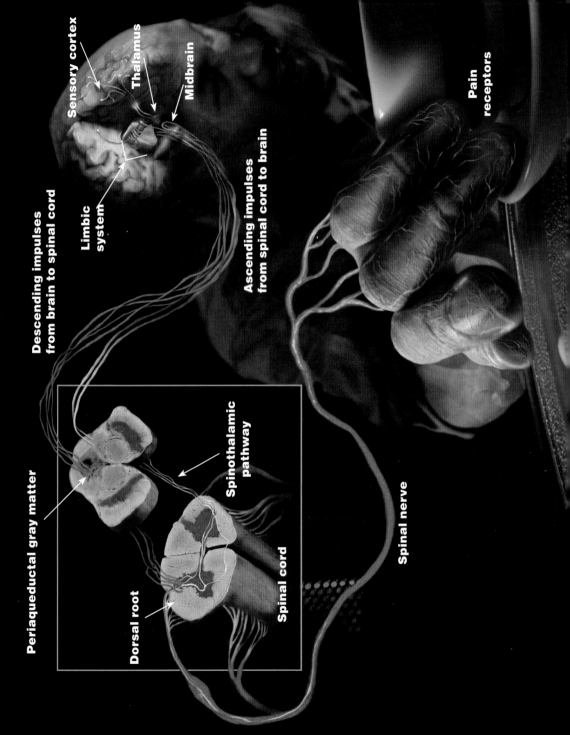

Sensory cortex

Thalamus

Midbrain

Limbic system

Descending impulses from brain to spinal cord

Ascending impulses from spinal cord to brain

Pain receptors

Periaqueductal gray matter

Spinothalamic pathway

Dorsal root

Spinal cord

Spinal nerve

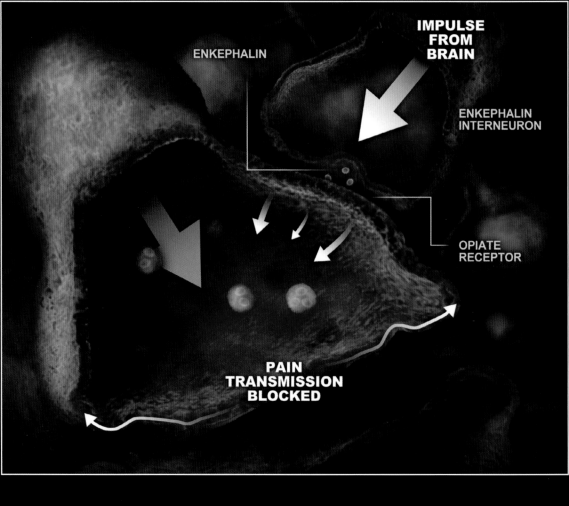

Figure 4: Cells in the medulla and the pons, when stimulated, release enkephalin (a morphine-like chemical) in the spinal cord and block the release of Substance P in the dorsal horn.

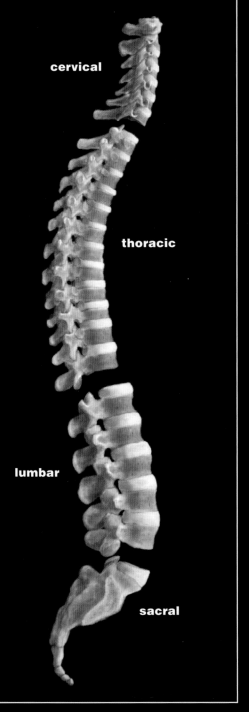

cervical

thoracic

lumbar

sacral

Figure 5: A side view of the spine.

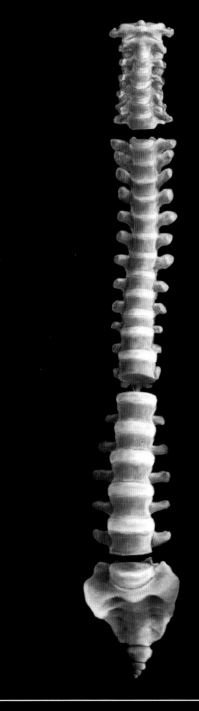

Figure 6: Frontal view of the spine.

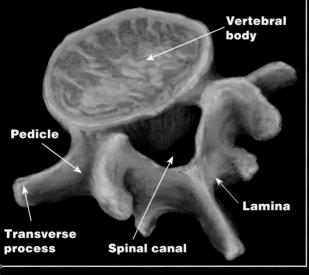

Figure 7: A normal lumbar vertebra.

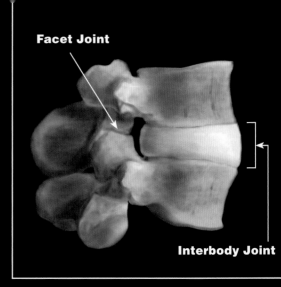

Figure 8: One of the body's joints.

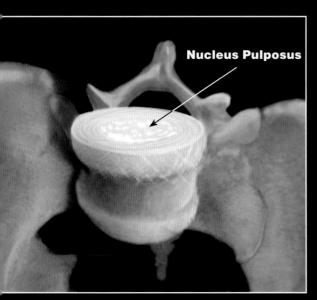

Figure 9: The nucleus pulposus

Figure 10: The annulus fibrosis

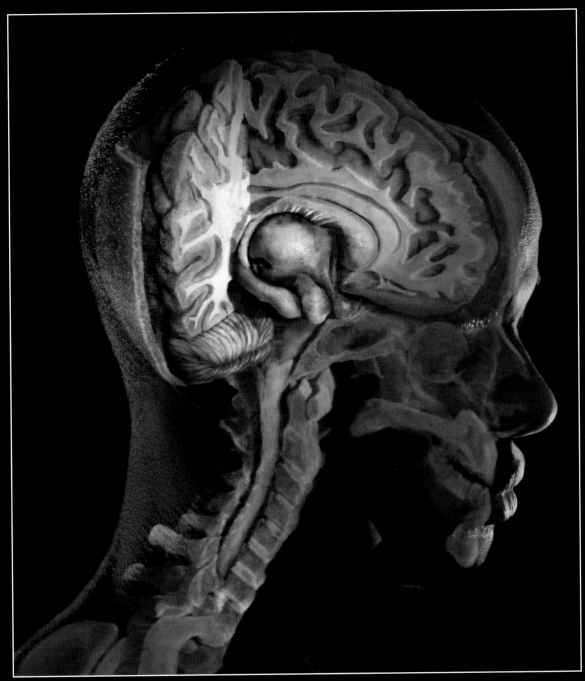

Figure 11: Here you can see the spinal cord and the brain, encased in bone.

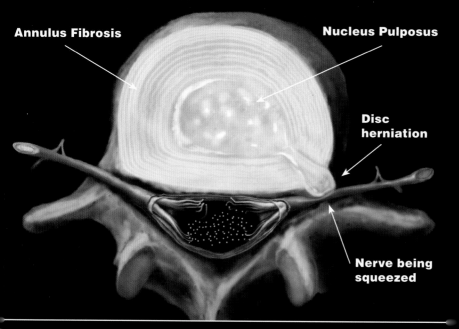

Annulus Fibrosis

Nucleus Pulposus

Disc herniation

Nerve being squeezed

Figure 12: Cross section of a herniated disc, squeezing a nerve root coming out of the spinal cord through the intervertebral foramen, causing pain down the leg.

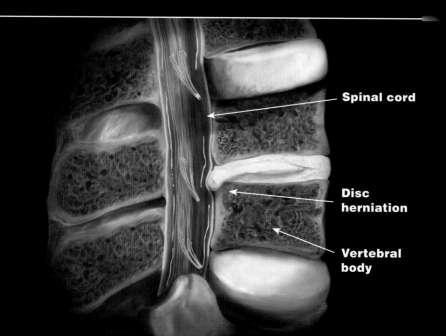

Spinal cord

Disc herniation

Vertebral body

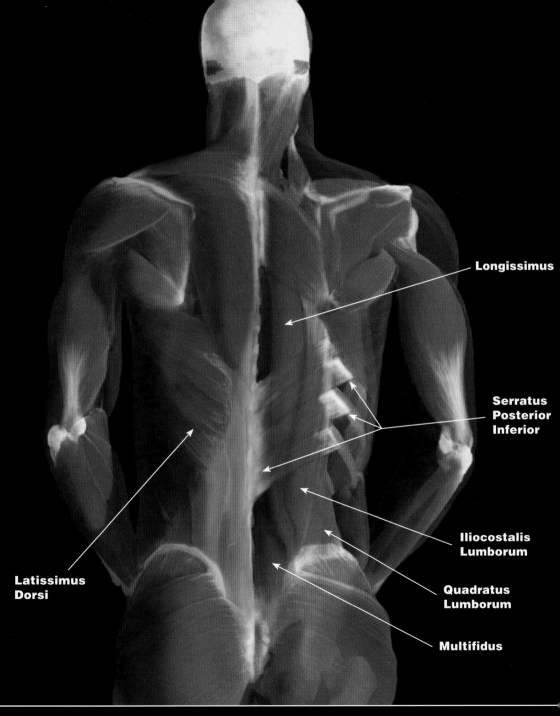

Longissimus

Serratus Posterior Inferior

Iliocostalis Lumborum

Quadratus Lumborum

Latissimus Dorsi

Multifidus

Figure 14: Some muscles that can cause back pain.

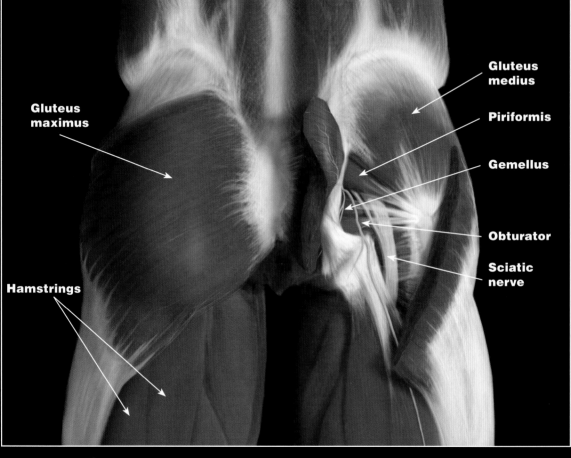

Figure 15: Muscles of the buttock and upper thigh.

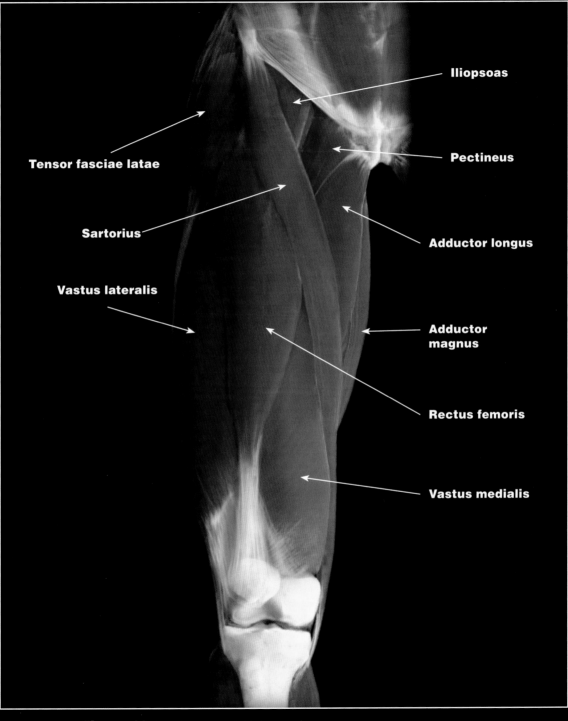

Figure 16: Frontal view of thigh muscles.

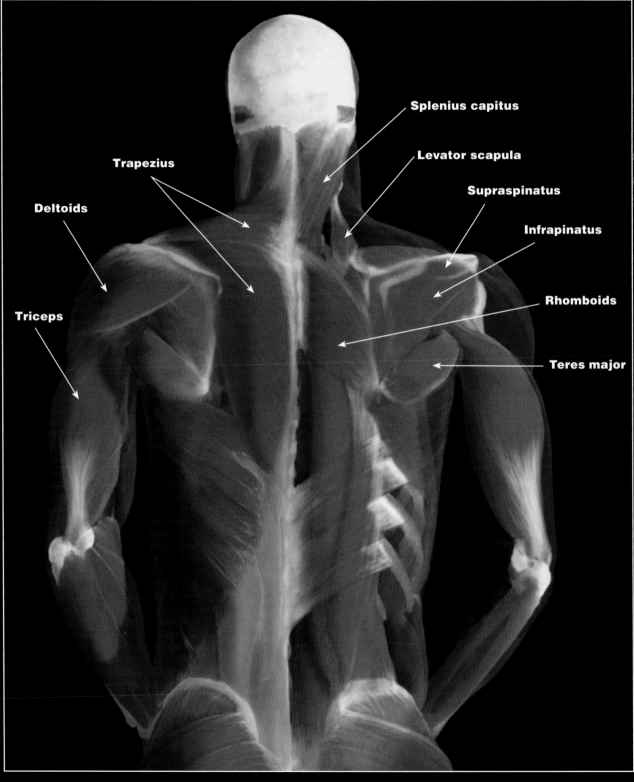

Figure 17: Upper back muscles.

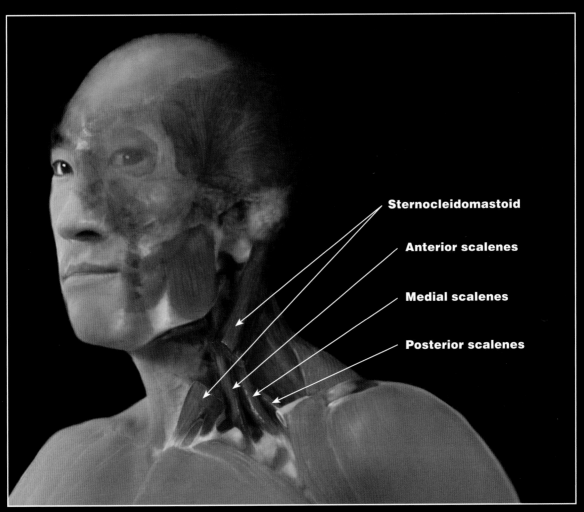

Figure 18: Neck and head muscles.

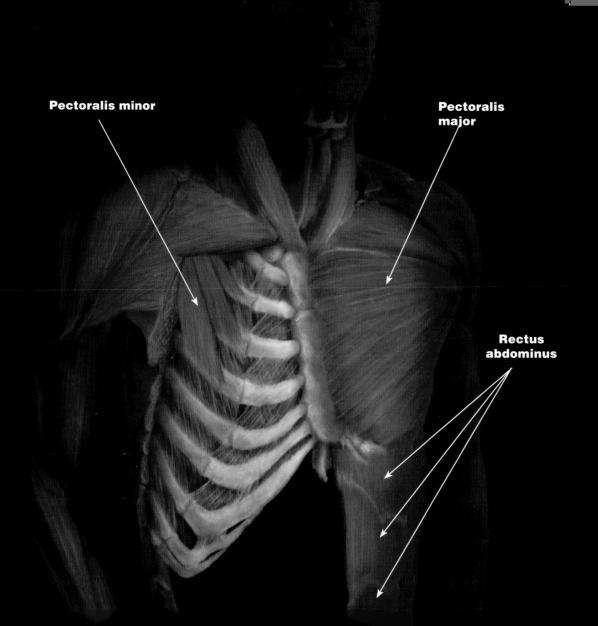

Pectoralis minor

Pectoralis major

Rectus abdominus

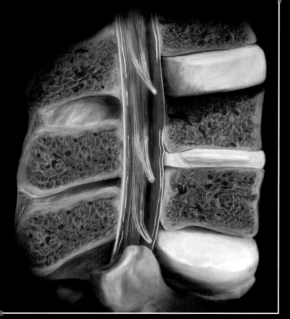

Figure 20: Degenerated, flattened disc.

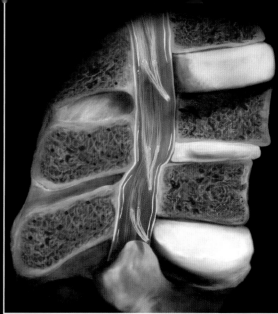

Figure 21: Spondylolisthesis (one vertebra overlapping another) and a flattened disc.

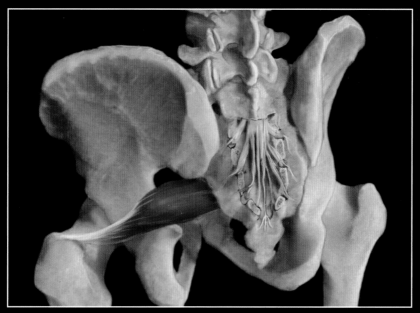

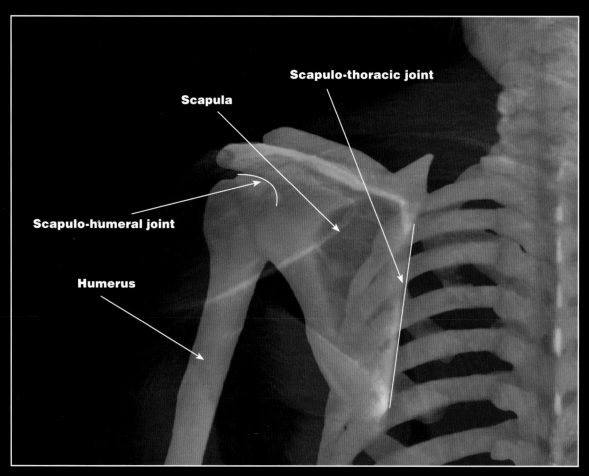

Figure 23: Anatomy of the shoulder.

6. REACHING

Lie on your back, with your arms at your sides and your legs extended on the mat. Breathe in deeply through your nose as you bring your right arm straight out from your body. When your arm is fully extended, exhale and bring it back across your chest to touch your left arm and as far as you can beyond the left arm. Then bring your arm back to the starting position and let go. Do this two more times, and then do the same movement three times with your left arm.

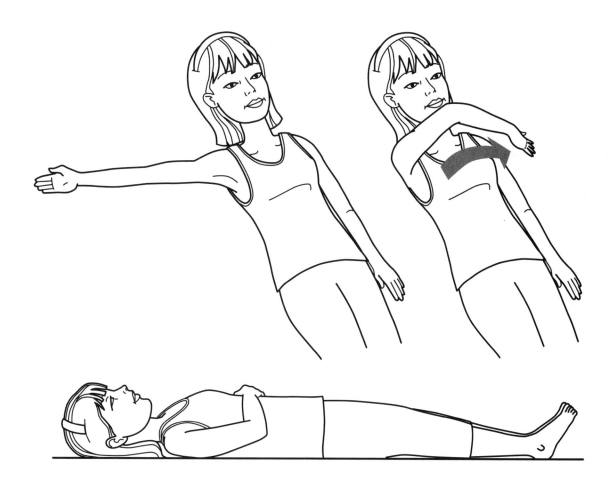

7. SHOULDER ROTATION

If you feel relatively flexible in your upper body, you can do this exercise with both arms at the same time. If there is significant stiffness, do it one arm at a time. Lie on your back, with your legs extended on the mat. Bring your arms, bent at the elbows, out from your sides so that your upper arms are at a 90-degree angle with your body. Then bend each elbow so that your forearm is straight up in the air also at a 90-degree angle. While keeping these 90-degree angles, move your forearms back so that your bent arms reach toward the mat and the backs of your hands touch the mat. If you cannot touch the mat, you have a deficit in external rotation.

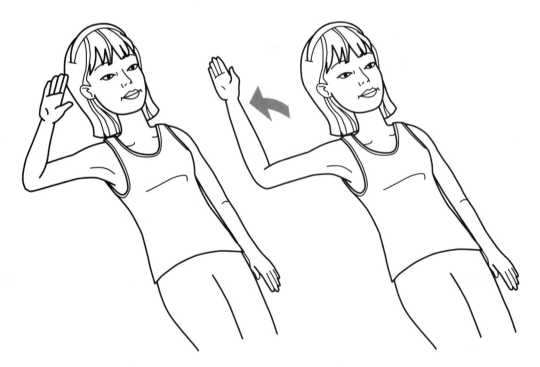

Now breathe in deeply through your nose and bring your forearms back up to 90 degrees. Breathe out slowly while you move your palms forward and down so that they are touching the mat. If you cannot touch the mat with your palms, you have a deficit in internal rotation.

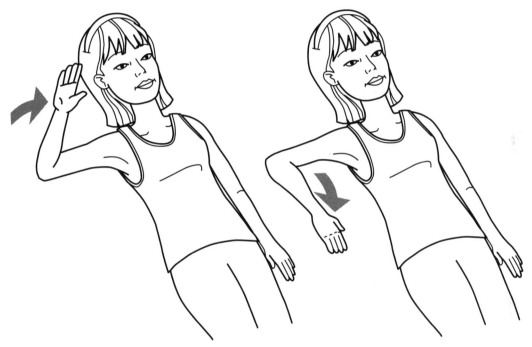

In this exercise, it is important to keep your shoulders flat on the mat when you are attempting to touch the mat with your palms. Do this exercise two more times.

This is generally the hardest of the upper body exercises because many patients with shoulder and neck pain have some deficit in internal rotation. But as you continue to do this exercise, you will see a gradual increase in the range of motion of both rotations.

8. SHOULDER FORWARD FLEX

As with the shoulder rotation, you can do this exercise with both arms at the same time if you feel relatively flexible in your upper body, or one arm at a time if there is significant stiffness when you attempt the movement.

Lie on your back, with your legs extended on the mat. Breathe in deeply through your nose. Breathe out slowly as you raise your arms up in the air, keeping your elbows straight, and then backward above your head so that your hands touch the mat. Breathe in as you bring your arms back to the starting position.

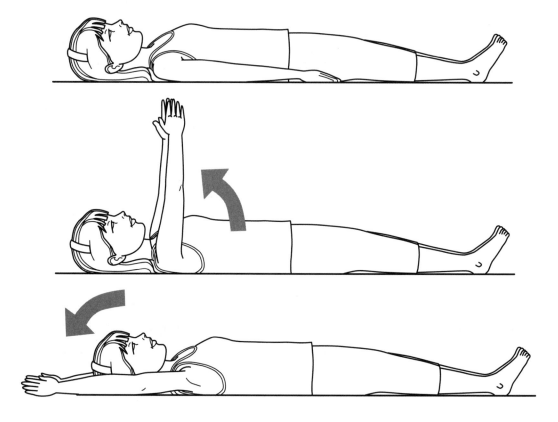

Do this exercise three times, and then do all the exercises in reverse order.

CHAPTER 12

Pregnancy and Back Pain

If we pay attention to our diet and remain physically active, our adult bodies do not change significantly, except under two conditions: during pregnancy and when we grow older, particularly after the age of fifty. Both will affect all the tissues in our body and increase the incidence and severity of back pain.

Let's look first at pregnancy.

You're pregnant. You've waited for this wonderful moment in your life. A new chapter is about to be written. There is so much to think about, and along with the excitement are all the concerns of an expectant mother. Will the baby be healthy? Will you be a good mother? Can you afford all that you want to do in your life? Will you work? Should you work?

Add to this the changes caused by hormones during pregnancy. They increase the flexibility of the ligaments, which gives you greater movement of the joints in the pelvis and low back, making it easier for the baby to enter the world. The hormones also alter mood, add weight and bloat, cause fatigue, and make sleeping difficult. All these changes and emotional stressors can contribute to low back pain and pelvic girdle pain.

Studies in the United States and Europe show that approximately 70 percent of pregnant women experience low back pain, and approximately one-third of them suffer from severe pain. The pain tends to increase throughout the pregnancy, and it can interfere with enough force to stop a woman from working. The pain is believed to be the result of multiple progressive causes.

To compensate in part for the added weight and displacement of the enlarging uterus, the normal curve of the spine in the low back increases, and the ligaments become more flexible and swollen from fluid retention. However, if you have kept the muscles in your lower body flexible and strong through exercise before you became pregnant, you can compensate for the potential problems associated with increased joint flexibility. A study shows that women who exercise before pregnancy are ten times more likely to continue to exercise regularly during pregnancy, and this definitely helps to eliminate or alleviate low back pain. After all, one of the main points of this book, if not *the* main point, is that exercise to keep your muscles healthy should always be on your to-do list, pregnant or not.

Although weight gain has not statistically been a factor in predicting which women will develop back pain during pregnancy, overweight women were less likely to participate in exercise during pregnancy. Women who gain more than twenty-four pounds by the thirtieth week of pregnancy appear to have an increased chance of back pain. Excessive weight before pregnancy is also a significant risk factor for premature birth, pregnancy-induced hypertension, pregnancy-related diabetes, and overweight babies.

Back pain during pregnancy is generally divided into two categories: low back pain and pelvic girdle pain. Low back pain refers to pain occurring from the twelfth rib down to the bottom of the buttock, where the buttock attaches to the thigh (iliac fold). Pelvic girdle pain is pain occurring from the top of the hip bone down to the iliac fold and typically in the region of the sacroiliac joint. In addition, the pain sometimes radiates to the back of the thigh and occurs at the same time or separately in the center of the pubic region, where the right and left pubic bones come together in the pubic symphysis. Pelvic girdle pain is thought to be related to increased and altered movement in the joints of the pelvis as pregnancy advances. Approximately 20 percent of pregnant women get pelvic girdle pain, and it is most often found in women with a history of low back pain and/or previous injury to the pelvis.

There are no studies in the medical literature on preventing back and pelvic girdle pain during pregnancy, but a variety of interventions have been used to treat it. We will use low back pain to stand for both low back pain and pelvic girdle pain in the rest of this chapter.

The American College of Obstetrics and Gynecology is supportive of exercise throughout pregnancy, albeit with certain precautions. It recommends thirty minutes a day of physical activity, such as walking, cycling (simulated by lying down in the later stages), swimming, and other forms of aerobics. As with a non-pregnant woman, a proper warm-up and cooldown before and after exercise are important. Exercise involving physical contact, the risk of falling, scuba diving, and high altitudes should be avoided. As pregnancy advances, you will have to modify your exercise routine.

There is controversy surrounding the effects of exercise on the fetus. Some studies suggest that vigorous physical activity could result in preterm delivery, prolonged labor, and reduced birth weight. A 2010 review of the literature on aerobic exercise during pregnancy concluded that regular exercise improved physical fitness for the mother, but it was unable to state definitively if there were specific risks or benefits for the infant. Let your common sense prevail. Reasonable amounts of exercise help you maintain feelings of well-being, tend to keep blood pressure normal, and serve as a deterrent to pregnancy-related diabetes—all important to pregnant women.

"Every woman who exercises while pregnant should monitor her body's reaction for unusual symptoms," advises Dixie L. Thompson, director of the Center for Physical Activity & Health at the University of Tennessee, Knoxville. "The following are signs that signal you should stop exercise and consult with your physician: vaginal bleeding or loss of amniotic fluid, unusual shortness of breath, dizziness or severe headaches, chest pain, muscle weakness, and painful uterine contractions. These are very rare occurrences, and women with healthy pregnancies usually will not encounter these or other complications. A helpful screening tool can be found online for safe exercise during pregnancy, developed by the Canadian Society for Exercise Physiology (www.csep.ca). In addition, ACOG (The American College of Obstetrics and Gynecology) has excellent information available (www.acog.org). Regular physical activity is an important part of a healthy lifestyle. For the majority of women, pregnancy does not prevent them from living an active life."

As with all back pain patients, pregnant women should adhere to the following:

• Wear shoes with a low heel and good ankle and arch support.

• Pay attention to proper body mechanics. Lift with your thigh muscles, not your back, meaning don't bend over to lift but rather squat, keeping your back upright, and don't twist your spine. Instead turn your entire body to face the object you wish to grasp.

• Sit in a comfortable chair with your back erect and with good support in your low back: feel the chair cushioning your low back.

• Make sure your mattress is firm enough so that you do not see the impression of your body in the mattress in the morning when you get out of bed. A moderately firm mattress encourages some movement at night, in contrast to a soft mattress, which inhibits movement.

• Consider sleeping on your side with a pillow between your legs.

• Don't attempt to carry objects heavier than what you can handle comfortably.

• If you need help, ask for it.

In studies where pregnant women with back pain were given classes on body mechanics, managing tension and stressful situations, and personalized exercises, the vast majority significantly reduced their pain during and after pregnancy. It is universally agreed that your pregnancy should involve some form of exercise, with proper precautions. It is recommended that you do not spend more than five to ten minutes in continuous exercise on your back after the third trimester, because in that position your enlarged uterus can inhibit blood flow back to the heart.

The exercises in Chapter 10 alternate positions so that you are not continuously on your back. Always check with your obstetrician before doing any exercises. If you have difficulties doing any of the exercises as your pregnancy progresses, modify or eliminate them.

Two additional interventions that have been studied and appear to reduce pain and/or discomfort are acupuncture and a specialized pillow for sleep. In a systematic review of acupuncture for low back pain, based on treatment of one hundred thousand patients in the United States, the United Kingdom, and Sweden, women reported better pain relief with acupuncture than with group physical therapy, and on the whole had no serious or lasting side effects. Also, the Ozzlo pillow, a hollowed-out pillow shaped like a nest for the abdomen, improved the sleep of pregnant women compared to a standard pillow. Unfortunately, this well-studied pillow appears not to be commercially available at the time of this writing. Newer pillows, such as the Boppy, Snoogle, and Leachco pillows, are commercially available, but to date, there are no published studies demonstrating their effectiveness.

BACK PAIN AFTER PREGNANCY

Women with a history of low back pain are more likely to have back pain during and after pregnancy. Even though back pain can persist after delivery, it usually improves for most women by the third month postpartum. After that, more women continue to report major reductions in pain, but after six months, the numbers appear to level off. Even so, if you still have back pain, do not despair. Why? Because women who are not free of pain at six months will continue to report the disappearance of pain over time, with improvement reported as late as four years after giving birth. Studies of women treated for back pain during pregnancy reveal that those at high risk for back pain are no more likely to suffer back pain than low-risk women, provided that they are informed about the risk and learn to exercise properly.

All the successful studies of the benefits of exercise in new mothers provided individualized exercises slowly over a long period of time to address the specific pain and needs of each mother. This was in contrast to failed studies, where all of the new mothers received the same exercise programs. Also, the studies showed that being evaluated prior to starting exercise and being observed at least every one to two weeks resulted in a better chance of success. The bottom line is that your chance of success with exercise is best with more supervision, frequency, intensity, and with a greater duration for the program that you participate in.

However, the best type of exercise has not yet been determined. Weak muscles appear to be associated not only with back pain but also with the inability to control urine and feces. Postpartum incontinence has been shown to be reduced by as much as 50 percent with exercises to strengthen the pelvic floor, such as squeezing the muscles in the region of the vagina and rectum. In contrast, teaching exercises to women who had no low back pain before and during pregnancy had no effect on whether or not they suffered persistent postpartum low back pain. In this group, it seems that alterations in ligaments and joint position associated with pregnancy may outweigh any muscle contributions to the pain. In the months following delivery, when hormones and ligaments return to baseline conditions, their pain will be gone in most cases.

The bottom line is that you will probably have back pain during and/or after your pregnancy, but you can minimize its frequency and/or intensity by understanding and paying attention to what causes the pain. Get in the habit of exercising and remaining trim before pregnancy, and once you are pregnant, modify your activities to minimize those things that will produce low back pain, and learn exercises that you can continue to do as your pregnancy progresses.

CHAPTER 13

Back Home with the Baby

Now that you're back home with your baby, I want you to take an honest assessment of yourself.

First of all, pregnancy puts significant stress on your low back muscles and also weakens the abdominal muscles by stretching them. At the risk of repeating myself, it is critical that you regain your normal weight by starting an exercise program that includes proper strengthening of your key postural muscles, particularly the abdominal muscles. If you do not, back pain may persist or begin.

If you are breastfeeding, pay attention to your posture. There is less strain on your back muscles if you bring the baby to the breast, not the breast to the baby. Another example is bending over the side of the crib to lift the baby. Don't do it. Instead lower the side of the crib so that you can lift the baby and bring it close to your body. It is the same situation when lifting the baby up from the floor: do not bend over to lift the baby. Instead bend your knees to the level of the baby, bring the baby to your body, and then straighten your legs. Twisting while bending places the most strain on your body. Remember our discussion about lifting with the legs, and not with the back? This is still very important.

Now, let's see how we can help your child. Kids learn by imitation. Are you or the father overweight? (See page 178 for definitions and discussion of diet and obesity.) Are either or both of you obese? Sixty-seven percent of Americans are overweight, sad to say, and 50 percent of them are actually obese. If you have a problem, so does your child. A child with one obese parent has a 50 percent chance of becoming obese. If both parents are obese, the likelihood jumps to 80 percent. Obesity in children commonly shows itself by age five. Don't put your child at risk early on by propelling him or her into a life plagued by obesity-related asthma, back pain, type 2 diabetes, sleep apnea, high blood pressure, high cholesterol, and heart and respiratory problems—let alone ridicule, social discrimination, low self-esteem, and depression. Exercise and sound eating practices are essential for a healthy life, and they must begin when the baby comes home from the maternity ward. As Hans Kraus used to say, "Geriatrics starts in the cradle." Children who are physically active are more likely to stay active as adults. Exercise will help their physical and emotional health.

Don't imprison a baby in a playpen. Let him or her move around on the lawn or a clean floor so that the muscles get a workout. The urge to move is natural. Crawling around on all fours also builds muscles. As your child grows, don't let him or her become a couch potato. Let your child run, swim, hike, ride a bike, and, under supervision, climb fences and trees.

In today's technology-obsessed society, children are often watching more TV, playing video games, and sitting at computers. In other words, they are finding ways to entertain themselves in a sedentary position. It's important that you encourage your children to run around, play outside, and learn games to exercise their minds and their bodies. You may need to limit the time they spend watching TV or playing video games. If they do play video games, play the kinds that make them move around, such as Wii Sports. Encourage them to play after-school sports, especially in noncompetitive leagues. It is important for children to stay active outside of school, especially after sitting almost nonstop for six to eight hours a day.

Studies have shown that the most common cause for low back pain in adolescents is the same as in adults: sprains and strains, caused most often by overuse during competitive sports. Strains are the result of excessive pulling on muscles, while sprains result from excessive pulling on ligaments. There are several ways to prevent this from happening. First, it is important to warm up and cool down after vigorous exercise and participation in sports. Second, it is important not to push children too hard while they are playing sports. Encourage them to try their hardest, but if their bodies cannot handle running the extra mile or doing the extra jumps, then stop. Forcing them to put additional pressure on their bodies when they can't handle it can cause injury.

According to Jack Harvey, MD and Suzanne Tanner, MD in the journal *Sports Medicine:* "In the young athlete, factors predisposing to back injury include the growth spurt, abrupt increase in training intensity or frequency, improper technique, unsuitable sports equipment, and leg-length inequality. Poor strength of the back extensor and abdominal musculature, and inflexibility of the lumbar spine, hamstrings, and hip flexor muscles may contribute to chronic low back pain."

If children are injured, please allow them to take the time to heal properly. Studies have shown that there is no magical amount of time that determines when it is safe to return to normal activities. It is important not to rush children back to normal activities if they are still complaining of pain, swelling, and/or limited strength or range of motion.

When your child leaves for school, be certain that he or she wears a backpack correctly. Many youngsters will wear one for most of the day, but if heavily loaded and worn incorrectly, it will cause your child to hunch forward, leading to poor posture, under- and over-developed muscles, and back strain. When loading the backpack, distribute the weight evenly, with the heaviest books centered closest to the body. When putting on the backpack, your youngster should bend at the knees and place the two loops over each arm so that they rest on the shoulders. The backpack should never be put on by swinging it from one arm to the other. Also, it should never be carried on one shoulder. Avoid imbalance that can cause tingling, pressure marks, or pain.

In 1952, Hans Kraus sounded the alarm after he used the Kraus-Weber tests on more than five thousand American schoolchildren, ages six to sixteen, and then compared the results with those of three thousand of their counterparts in Austria, Switzerland, and Italy. He found that 58 percent of the American children failed one or more of the six tests, while only 9 percent of the European children failed one or more of the six tests. American kids fared poorly against other cultures that had not yet had the "advantages" of modern living. The Asia Foundation reported the same kind of lopsided results when compared to Pakistani youngsters, who tested far higher than the Americans. The same held true when researchers at Kyushu University tested six thousand Japanese youngsters. No one is immune from the effects of decreased physical activity. When the Austrian physician Dr. Willi Nagler conducted follow-up studies of Austrian schoolchildren years later (when modern conveniences were common), he found that the failure rate on the Kraus-Weber tests had nearly doubled.

Despite the obvious problems of our children, Kraus almost always met with opposition wherever he presented findings of the K-W tests and expressed the idea that not enough exercise was causing many ills. Both he and his concepts were considered "radical" and "unpatriotic" in medical circles. "This I found when my associates and I presented our findings at the 1955 annual meeting of the American Medical Association," Kraus reported in his 1965 book *Backache, Stress, and Tension,* adding that "most of the audience did not believe in exercise at all, and they were practically shouting at me when discussing my paper."

John B. Kelly, twice an Olympic gold medalist in rowing (best known to the public as the father of actress Grace Kelly), brought to the attention of President Dwight Eisenhower an article that Kraus wrote on exercising and deconditioning. It struck a nerve. When Eisenhower was the commanding general of American and British forces in Europe in World War II, he had been concerned about the high rate of rejection of recruits due to failure on their physical examination. Eisenhower invited Kraus to a special sports luncheon at the White House on July 11, 1955, and soon after established the President's Council for Physical Fitness.

It turned out, however, that the opposition Kraus had faced from other doctors paled in comparison with that of physical educators who joined against him. First, they managed to get the word "Physical" removed from the name of the council. It became the President's Council for Youth Fitness. This, Kraus said, ignored the point that "under-exercise threatens not only children but the entire adult population. Almost all of them [physical educators] regarded the idea of formal exercise as unpalatable. Instead they suggested various sports and games as an alternative. This sounds very well, but . . . some sports are better than others for physical conditioning, and some sports may even be harmful. The answer was and is basic exercise programs geared to the correction of muscular deficiencies and development of good hearts and lungs."

Shortly after this, Kraus attended a meeting of physical educators. He asked, "Why are you against exercise?" One answered for all. "Very simple," he said. "Twenty-five years ago, we gave exercises to schoolchildren. And as far as I'm concerned, that's enough. We were looked down on as the boobs of the school system. We had no status at all. So we changed our emphasis. Now we're not the boobs we used to be. We're respected members of the academic community. We are educators—physical educators if you wish. We're not 'exercise teachers' anymore. We're educators, coaches, and administrators. You want to know the truth? Exercise is finished! It's passé; it's out of date. You want us to turn back the clock. Well, I'm telling you, Doctor, we don't care what your findings show; we're not going back to the old days. We've worked hard to get where we are, and we are going to stay there."

Kraus replied, "From an athletic point of view, we have the most undemocratic schools in the world. The school can have as many as three to four thousand students, but the only ones who receive systematic muscular training are those who've won a place on one of the varsity athletic teams. This is contrary to common sense, which tells you that the children who are the least exercised are the ones who need it most. Instead of lavishing attention on the gifted athletes, schools should institute broad, noncompetitive exercise programs that benefit all the students. This does not mean that competitive sports should be neglected. Sports have their place, but that place comes after the physical needs of the overall student body have been met. That should be the aim of physical education."

Kraus advocated imaginative exercise programs, starting, for example, with bunny hops and cat crawls, followed by chinning, rope climbing, tumbling, and leapfrog, before taking on exercises that challenged strength, endurance, and coordination. "The more challenging they are, the more interesting they will be," he said. "A young child should learn to improve his abilities without actually competing with other children. He should measure his own improvement, not compare his performance with that of another. Children grow at different rates, and competition should come in later childhood—say, after twelve—and then competition should be encouraged only when it buds spontaneously. To force a young child to compete when the contest is hopeless and the child knows that he is destined to be a loser will do the child no good. There is nothing more disheartening to a youngster, and he falls into the lifelong habit of always doubting himself. Above all, the teachers should set the example. He or she should be fit, should come to class in gym clothes, and should work personally with the children. He should not only be able to do what they do, but he should be able to do any exercise better than they can." As an added bonus, "The exercise class can be used to teach discipline, an area which is neglected, if not ignored, in schools because it is usually confused with regimentation."

Probably because of Kraus, who was treating his back, President Kennedy changed the name back to the President's Council on Physical Fitness, later amended to the President's Council on Physical Fitness and Sports by President Lyndon Johnson. But no matter who was president, matters only got worse despite the best of publicized intentions. For example, on June 23, 2000, President Bill Clinton directed that the Secretary of Health and Human Services and the Secretary of Education work on "strategies to promote better health for our nation's youth through physical activity and fitness." He did this after receiving a report stating, "Our nation's young people are, in large measure, inactive, unfit, and increasingly overweight. In the long run, this physical inactivity threatens to reverse the decades-long progress we have made in reducing deaths from cardiovascular diseases and to devastate our national health care budget. In the short run, physical inactivity has contributed to an unprecedented increase in childhood obesity that is currently plaguing the United States." The national health objectives for the decade 2010–20 promote participation in physical activity and sports among young people as a critical national priority.

President Barack Obama has changed the name of the council to the President's Council on Fitness, Sports and Nutrition, and First Lady Michelle Obama is leading the "Let's Move" campaign that aims to reduce childhood obesity in the United States within a generation. The Let's Move website (www.letsmove.gov) offers helpful tips, strategies, and updates on combating obesity in children.

But far more is needed. Consider the 2010 *Shape of the Nation Report* on physical education:

- Only five states require physical education (PE) in every grade K–12.

- Only one state aligns with the nationally recommended 150 minutes per week of PE in elementary school and 225 minutes per week in middle and high school.

- More than half of all states (thirty-two) permit waivers and/or exemptions for students from taking PE, a 77 percent increase from 2006.

- Forty-eight states (94 percent) have their own state standards for physical education, but only thirty-four states (67 percent) require local districts to comply or align with these standards.

- Only nineteen states (37 percent) require some form of student assessment in physical education.

- Fewer states (fourteen versus twenty-two in 2006) require physical education grades to be included in students' grade point averages.

• Only thirteen states (25 percent) require schools to measure height and weight for each student.

We already have an epidemic.

We doubled our expenditures for health care from 1993 to 2007, from $3,468 to $7,421 per capita. However, more money spent is not making our system better. Though we are spending more on prevention, we continue to fall behind other countries that spend far less yet achieve greater longevity and health-related quality of life. Our resources need to be spent more wisely. The physical condition of our country's youths needs to be prioritized. Healthy habits of exercise and positive experiences in sports can improve the health and well-being of the next generation.

CHAPTER 14

Back Pain and Aging

The good news is that you can remain physically and mentally fit for as long as you live. When we're younger, nature helps most of us by giving us strong bodies that respond well to our needs as long as we live with healthy habits. With progressing age, however, it is even more important to have a healthy lifestyle because nature will start to let us down.

Studies in all Western societies show that as we get older, more people will report multiple longer-lasting pains. Chronic pain, which is defined as a pain that occurs almost daily and has lasted for more than three months, is reported by approximately 18 percent of adults younger than fifty-five and in multiple studies, the rates are 30 percent to 65 percent of adults between fifty-five and sixty-five. The percentage levels off and declines somewhat for seniors over eighty-five: 25 percent to 55 percent of them say they have chronic pain. It seems possible that elderly patients under-report their pain because they are resigned to it in the belief that pain is an inevitable part of aging. In any case, persistent pain has a negative impact on quality of life and is associated with increases in depression, anxiety, anger, and problems concentrating, sleeping, socializing, and just getting anything done.

The most frequent chronic pain in the elderly is in the leg (often related to arthritis in the knee or hip) and low back. Understanding back pain in the elderly is more challenging than in the younger populations. As we age, there is a natural decline in the structure and function of all of our organs. Even though we cannot prevent these changes, a healthy lifestyle can minimize them. Recognizing how our bodies age and becoming aware of the habits and activities that add to our decreased capacities can help us remain independent, active, and productive. Some of the important changes that occur in our bodies can be positively affected by choices you make each day.

OXIDATIVE STRESS

All of us, just like all other living creatures, have to burn fuel to produce energy to operate the systems that keep us alive and functioning. This process of energy production takes place in a part of the cell called the mitochondria. The mitochondria don't transform all the fuel to energy. The wasted parts—like smoke from a candle, the part of the candle that wasn't completely burned—are chemicals generically called oxidants; specifically, reactive oxygen species (ROS), otherwise known as free radicals. ROS are unstable, meaning that they will search for some tissue in the body with which they can combine. When they combine with part of a blood vessel, for example, or with cartilage, muscle, or fatty tissue, they cause some damage to that tissue. This process takes place throughout our lives and has a cumulative destructive effect on all the organs in our bodies. As we age, the mitochondria themselves are victims of free radicals and become progressively less efficient. This leads to an overall decrease in the energy we feel and in the physical power of our bodies. The reduced efficiency of the mitochondria is thought to contribute to the overall loss of the total number of cells in the body as we grow older. Although the number of mitochondria is thus reduced and their function impaired, physical activity can increase the actual number of mitochondria so that we can overcome some of the energy loss we may experience as we age.

We also produce compounds called antioxidants that prevent ROS from doing damage. Studies have shown that foods containing carotenoids, the compounds that create the red, yellow, and orange colors of fruits and vegetables, and are also found in many dark green vegetables, the antioxidant vitamins C and E, and coenzyme Q10 (CoQ10) all appear to help maintain muscle strength and protect against the destructive effects of free radicals.

SPECIFIC ORGAN CHANGES AND BACK PAIN

Structures in the spine change with age. All of the variations of the spine that were described in Chapter 5 will tend to grow more pronounced as we get older. For example, the discs between the vertebrae lose their water content and shrink, accounting for the fact that Grandpa and Grandma are getting shorter. The cartilage that lines the joints becomes frayed and may allow bone to touch bone, which can be painful and limit motion. Myelin, the fatty material that covers our nerves, may thin, decreasing the nerves' ability to transmit sensations, impairing older folks' balance and increasing their chances of falling and injuring themselves. But just as in the younger age groups, the mere presence of a nerve diagnosis or of some specific change in the body may not explain a pain complaint. Many back pain patients I have seen, with prior diagnoses of nerve problems such as neuropathies (abnormal functioning of the nerves) related to diabetes and HIV, had treatable muscle pain.

MUSCLES AND AGING

Muscles tend to get smaller, weaker, and less efficient as we age, a condition referred to as *sarcopenia*. It literally means "poverty of flesh," analogous to the well-known *osteopenia*—thinning of bone that is not yet severe enough to be labeled *osteoporosis*. Muscles in individuals over the age of sixty-five are found to have fewer muscle fibers and a decreased ability of those fibers to contract quickly. Taken together, this reduces our maximum strength and ability to respond quickly as we age. For example, male weightlifters over the age of sixty can lift a maximum weight 30 percent less than lifters in their twenties and thirties, with female lifters showing an even greater decline.

MUSCLE INJURY AND REPAIR

Muscles are designed to deal with the inevitable damage that they suffer when we overuse or misuse them. Who hasn't lifted something too heavy and felt some sort of strain? For those of you who are athletes, it would be hard to believe that you never experienced some nagging pain while engaged in your sport. The pain was related to some degree of muscle injury, and the repair process, in most cases, eliminated the pain and allowed you to function fully again. Cells that rebuild your injured muscle are called satellite cells. These cells decrease significantly after the age of seventy, and, when exposed to stress at an older age, they die more easily than cells in younger individuals. The loss of satellite cells is thought to be one of the major reasons that our muscles shrink as we age.

The ongoing ability of the satellite cell to reproduce is based on the length of the tips of the chromosomes, called telomeres, which are thought to shorten with age and eventually disappear. This process accounts for the inability of certain cells, like muscles, to regenerate.

There is some good news, though. In animal experiments, when the satellite cells of older animals were placed into a younger animal, the cells acted as if they were young cells. Conversely, young cells placed into old rats acted like old cells. This suggests that the environment surrounding the cell is an important factor in how well it functions. In addition, experiments have shown that moderate exercise in elderly people can actually prevent shortening or can even lengthen the telomeres in satellite cells.

What is the environment for *your* muscles? A good environment has a rich blood supply that brings in adequate amounts of oxygen; enough energy produced by an abundance of efficient mitochondria; circulating nutrients in the blood, such as proper amounts of glucose (sugar), that have easy access into the cells; and healthy fats, known as high-density lipoproteins (HDLs), would predominate. If you are obese, chances are that your environment is not good for your muscles or for any of your tissues. The same holds true if you're not exercising regularly.

Forty-two percent of US adults over the age of seventy have metabolic syndrome, which is associated with a progressive decline in physical functioning and is defined as a combination of excessive fat in the abdominal area, high blood pressure, and in the blood: elevated levels of triglycerides (fats that are associated with high blood pressure, heart disease, and stroke), low levels of high-density lipoprotein (HDL) cholesterol (fats that protect our bodies), and elevated blood sugar.

MUSCLE FUNCTION

Muscles start to lose their ability to function after the age of forty. A number of changes take place. Muscle mass drops by 10 percent to 15 percent every ten years between the ages of fifty and seventy, and an additional 30 percent between the ages of seventy and eighty. The result is slower reaction times as well as the loss of overall strength associated with decreased muscle mass. Muscle fibers are connected to a nerve that tells them when and how much to contract or relax. The nerve and the muscle fibers together are called a *motor unit* (MU). MUs are composed of similar fibers of varying number so that the muscle may move strongly or slightly depending on the task. Different MUs are involved in using your hand and fingers to operate tweezers to remove a splinter than to lift a ten-pound weight. Both actions involve some of the same muscles but require very different amounts of force and nuances of movement. With aging, there is a reduction in the number of MUs. With loss of smaller MUs, a larger number of fibers will contract when a muscle is activated, resulting in the loss of fine motor skills. Decreased muscle mass results in decreased breaking down of glucose. If you haven't reduced your calorie intake, and you have less muscle mass, you will gain weight. You may notice people over sixty who are not overweight. I guarantee that they are consuming fewer calories than they did when they were fifty.

OBESITY AND PAIN

The United States and most industrialized countries are faced with an epidemic of obesity that affects all age groups but exerts its most harmful effects in the elderly. Excessive weight is associated with chronic pain and disability, as well as diabetes, high blood pressure, arthritis, and heart disease. The measure that is most often used in the medical literature to define excess weight is called the body mass index, better known as BMI. The BMI is calculated by dividing your weight in kilograms by your height in meters squared: BMI=

weight in KG/height^2 (in meters). There are charts that you can find online where you can just plug in the numbers in pounds and inches and get your BMI. One is the National Institutes of Health BMI calculator at www.nhlbisupport.com/bmi. A BMI greater than 27.3 for men and 27.8 for women is considered overweight; 30 to 34.9 for both is considered obese; and 35 or more is considered severely obese.

Obesity, particularly in the abdominal area, appears to be a very important factor on its own. In one large multiyear study, elderly obese patients were twice as likely to have chronic pain as the normal-weight individuals, and severely obese patients were four times as likely to have it. The most common pains, as you might have guessed, were in the low back, the knee, and the hip.

THE SOLUTION

EXERCISE

Even though we're not going to have the strength and endurance of a twenty-year-old when we're seventy, studies show that individuals who exercise function at a much higher level than those who don't. Elite athletes will notice a decrease in performance after forty but are still able to compete into their eighties. One study showed that an eighty-five-year-old weightlifter could lift as much as a nonexercising sixty-five-year-old. But, clearly, you don't have to be an accomplished athlete to benefit from exercise.

Numerous studies have shown that regular exercise retards the progression of age-related skeletal muscle loss and weakness. Two types of exercise were studied: endurance training, referring to the ability to continue toward the completion of a physically demanding task; and resistance training, which is another way to say strengthening exercise. As you might guess, the effects are different for the two types of exercise. Endurance training will increase both the number of mitochondria in your body and the blood supply to the muscles, as well as improve heart function. Resistance training will generally increase muscle mass, strength, and power. The combination is just what the doctor ordered. If you have pain and have become weak, resistance exercise, such as lifting weights, may not be possible. The good news is that recent studies have shown that you can build new muscle by doing endurance exercise training, such as riding a stationary bike. Because our older bodies do not respond as quickly to the effects of exercise, it is important to be committed for the long haul when you begin your exercise routine. Don't be surprised or disappointed if you can't exercise every day at the start. Do what you can and remember that the first two weeks are the hardest. After that, if you exercise at least every other day, you will see an improvement in your energy and greater ease in doing exercises. As important as regular exercise is, it is only part of the formula to maintain your vitality as you age.

CALORIE RESTRICTION

Just look around, and it is obvious that far too many Americans (as well as individuals in most Western countries) eat too much and are overweight. We are faced with an obesity epidemic. Obesity is associated with pain and disease. What is interesting and hopeful, however, is the recognition that restricting calories over time can actually prevent disease and aging. Initial studies on rats showed that a balanced diet that restricted calories produced healthier, longer-living animals.

These same findings were duplicated in a seventeen-year study of monkeys. The monkeys were divided into two groups. One group received 30 percent fewer calories than the normally fed group. The calorie-restricted group had minimal loss of muscle mass, no diabetes, and reduced incidences of hypertension and brain atrophy compared to the higher-calorie group. Although animal studies aren't always applicable to humans, for me, it's a no-brainer! Eating a lower-calorie, balanced diet will decrease obesity and a variety of diseases. It will also help maintain muscle mass, your ability to be physically and mentally fit, and help prolong your life.

QUALITIES OF THOSE WHO LIVE TO BE ONE HUNDRED

Studies of people who are one hundred years old or more and live healthy, productive lives reveal three major traits:

1. Ability to accept loss. If we live long enough, we will all lose someone we love: a parent, friend, spouse. Accepting life on life's terms and going forward may not be easy, but it is worth the struggle.

2. A sense of humor. Acceptance of others' irritating habits and behaviors and being able to see the charming qualities of the people in our lives reduces stress and allows us the pleasure of being alive each day. Experiencing life as struggle and stress is associated with shortened telomeres.

3. A passion for something. Using our minds is like using our muscles. If you don't use it, you lose it. Creativity can be your gift if you invest your time in things, projects, plans, and people that inspire you. It's never too late to engage in a new or ignored interest.

MANAGING BACK PAIN

You or someone you know is getting older and struggling with back pain. You may have been told that you have a problem in your spine that is causing your pain. Young or old, the most common cause of back pain is muscles. Although the findings on your imaging *may* be the reason for your pain, chances are that muscles are causing some or all of your discomfort. After learning about the effects of age in causing low back pain, you want to exercise and avoid gaining excessive weight, but you're having a hard time because every time you try to exercise, your pain gets worse.

Here is a patient who had a complicated problem and found relief with our exercises. I will call him Herb. He is an eighty-four-year-old married architect with pain in his mid and low back that radiated to the right hip and thigh. He described this as an intermittent aching, stabbing, shooting sensation, made worse by sitting for more than thirty minutes, standing for more than fifteen minutes, or walking.

Herb's pain began eight years before he saw me. He noticed a stooping tendency when he stood up. This tendency increased for the next three years. When he tried to stand up straight, he would feel discomfort in his midback. Herb was involved in a motor vehicle accident five years before seeing me, which increased his low back pain. Imaging studies showed degeneration of all the discs in his lower spine and some narrowing of the canal. A neurologist noticed that some of the muscles in his lower body were smaller than expected, and he thought this suggested that Herb had contracted polio when he was a youngster.

His examination was interesting. It showed something that I see frequently: good strength in his muscles that hold him up straight (postural muscles), but stiffness in his low back muscles and his hamstrings (muscles in the back of his thighs), so that he could hardly bend over with his knees straight when I asked him to touch his toes. When lying down, he could not raise his left leg more than 60 degrees and his right leg 40 degrees. Herb was taught all twenty-one exercises found in Chapter 10. His flexibility improved, and in four weeks his pain was gone. Three years later, when I last checked in with him, Herb was continuing his exercises and was pain free.

STEP CARE

Herb could have undergone a variety of treatments, including surgery, nerve blocks, and strong pain medication. All of these treatments may or may not have reduced his symptoms to some degree, but all would have had potentially unwanted side effects. In any case, Herb had very stiff muscles. Treating those stiff muscles relieved his pain and returned him to an active, comfortable, productive life. He received the simplest, cheapest, least harmful treatment directed at the most common cause of pain and stiffness: muscle. Rational care of any medical condition should be guided by *step care,* which is pursuing first the intervention that is potentially most effective and least expensive. If that doesn't work, go to the next step. In this case, the only way that Herb would ever have been helped would be to examine his muscles for strength and flexibility using a simple-to-use and easily reproducible test that you took in Chapter 9. The Kraus-Weber test should be part of any examination performed to understand why you have back pain.

If you have not exercised recently or ever, you can still be helped. Our exercises can change your life for the better. They are created to produce the minimal needed strength and flexibility in your major muscles that hold you upright. Once you have mastered the Kraus-Marcus exercises and can pass the K-W tests, you can then add other exercises to satisfy your personal needs. Pay attention to the exercise guidelines we covered at the bottom of page 61. Studies have shown that even regular walking counts as exercise, because it will have many of the same effects as other exercises. Whatever you do, start slowly. Never do more than you can handle comfortably to start and slowly increase the amount and difficulty of your exercise. Always warm up first and cool down at the end. Remember Herb. Strength isn't the whole story; flexibility counts. Never give up.

Make the commitment to yourself and have the integrity to do what you are promising. You are the only one who can make this part of your life better. There is nothing more important. I know that if you do your exercises every day, you will see significant improvement within three months in your strength, energy, mood, and sleep. You have nothing to lose.

CHAPTER 15

Dieting

The most effective weight loss diet is the Guatemalan Chicken Soup with Maui Pickled Prickly Pear diet. *Joking!* After doing my homework on which diet is best to lose weight, I found the answer to be what common sense and my wife have been telling me for years: eat fewer calories, and you will lose weight. It doesn't matter what kind of calories you eat. If the total number is less than what you've been eating, you will lose weight as long as you maintain your activity level. A landmark study of 811 motivated, overweight adults, funded by the National Institutes of Health (NIH), found that reduced-calorie diets result in significant weight loss, period. Regardless of the percentages of calories from fat, protein, and carbohydrates, all participants who consistently attended the scheduled support group sessions regularly lost the most weight, and all participants who completed the experiment lost on average approximately ten pounds in one year.

Approximately 20 percent of the weight loss for the first year was regained in the second year, with an overall trend suggesting that without regular encouragement from weight-loss-savvy professionals, much of the lost weight would be regained. This is both an encouraging and foreboding finding. All we need to do is reduce the amount of calories we consume, but most of us who are overweight do not seem to be able to maintain a reduced-calorie diet or the weight loss we achieved.

If even a motivated group of individuals could not maintain any reduced-calorie diet, is there any hope? Yes. But, it appears, only if you have some form of help. An exciting 2000 study from France, which is now being replicated in more than one hundred towns in Europe, addressed the obesity epidemic in children. Recognizing the failure of all attempts to encourage weight reduction in their children, two small towns marshaled the cooperation of everyone—from the mayor to schoolteachers, doctors, pharmacists, caterers, restaurant owners, sports associations, the media, scientists, and various branches of town government—to encourage children to eat lower-calorie meals and to become more physically active. Gymnasiums and playgrounds were built. Areas were set aside for walking trails, and sports instructors were hired. Families were offered workshops to teach them how to cook nutritionally, and high-risk families were offered counseling.

A follow-up study—"Ensemble Prévenons l'Obésité des Enfants" (EPODE), or, in English, "Together We Can Prevent Obesity in Children"—showed that it worked. The prevalence of overweight children had fallen to 8.8 percent compared to surrounding towns where the prevalence was 17.8, which was similar to the national trend. It appears that none of us struggling with our weight can overcome the problem easily on his or her own. There are too many messages encouraging us to eat poorly and too few opportunities to be physically active. Unless something changes (imagine a total commitment of an entire community, as in the EPODE study), obesity rates will continue to rise, and the number of surgical procedures to control obesity will continue to increase.

Although calorie reduction results in weight loss, some diets appear to be better than others when it comes to lowering bad cholesterol. Obesity is related to higher levels of cholesterol. We generally look at three types of cholesterol: high-density lipoproteins, known as HDLs, or the "good" cholesterol, which actually reduce the buildup of cholesterol deposits in blood vessels known as plaque; low-density lipoproteins, known as LDLs; and triglycerides. The latter two are "bad" cholesterol and are associated with heart disease, stroke, and high blood pressure.

Popular diets, such as the Atkins diet, that prescribe low amounts of carbohydrates (foods that contain sugar and those that come from wheat such as bread, pasta, and pastries) and high amounts of animal protein (beef, pork, poultry, eggs, and dairy products) are found to lower weight and cholesterol. This was an interesting observation because common wisdom said that eating a lot of animal protein, which also contains animal fat, should raise your cholesterol. The Atkins-type diets lowered cholesterol more than diets high in carbohydrate and low in protein and fat, but they did not lower the bad cholesterol, LDLs. An important study done in 2009 showed that if you substituted plant protein (nuts, soy, beans) for animal protein, the problem was solved: LDLs were also reduced. So if you can enjoy eating proteins from plant products, your most effective diet for addressing any cholesterol problem is high plant protein, low carbohydrate.

So many of us have been told to lose weight, and have tried without success. Why is it so difficult to succeed? There may be genetic and hormonal reasons. And some medications may be associated with weight gain, (such as many antidepressants). But three factors that are in your control can easily be addressed:

1. Increase your physical activity. If you never walk anywhere, start to do that. If you walk two blocks a day, increase it to four. If you go to the gym once a week, increase it to twice a week. The idea is to begin where you

are now and increase slowly and steadily. Don't take on more than you can handle, but work your way up. Make yourself a winner by taking on an achievable goal.

2. Don't attempt total deprivation. Avoid starvation diets. Your body senses that you are starving, and it adjusts by slowing your metabolism, the rate at which calories are burned. This makes it harder to lose weight. Being able to lose weight and maintain the loss requires changing the way you eat and increasing physical activity. Just as you changed your activity level gradually, do the same with diet. In other words, start slowly. Make one simple change. I recommend to my patients that they stop eating bread and pastries. Some love bread and can't imagine living without it. They soon learn, though, that after a short while, the craving for bread diminishes and their weight starts to drop. Then stop eating pasta or only allow it (and bread) as a treat; let's say on Sundays.

3. Learn how many calories are in the food that you eat. When patients tell me that all they eat is salad, but they're gaining weight, I have to remind them that any sauce or dressing may contain high-calorie ingredients. When you are out at a restaurant, it is best to avoid foods that may hide unwanted calories.

If you are not familiar with the number of calories in everything that you eat, start with getting yourself a calorie book to know what you take in and then let your conscience be your guide.

Some of you have struggled with weight for your entire lives, even before you had back pain. You can't remember being thin. Although losing weight will be more of a challenge for you, do not despair. You can win this battle, but not overnight. You may not be ready to commit to weight loss yet. You may be thinking, "I have lost so much. Now you ask me to give up one of the few pleasures I can still have?" If you're not ready to do a total diet makeover, see if you can choose one modified area—like no bread on weekdays—but stick to it. When you're ready, add another modified area. You didn't gain the weight overnight, or, in most cases, lose your ability for physical activities overnight. Don't expect to lose the weight quickly. Weight lost slowly and steadily is more likely to stay off. Most important is to first admit that there is a problem making your pain and quality of life worse.

CHAPTER 16

Drugs, Vitamins, Supplements, and Snake Oil

C hances are that your odyssey of back pain (your own or perhaps a loved one's) has exposed you to traditional and/or alternative medications. When you turn on the television, open the newspaper or health magazine, or walk the aisles of your drugstore or vitamin shop, you will be exposed to the variety of drugs, vitamins, and minerals that promise to ease your pain. For simplicity, I will use the word *drugs* to mean all of the things we put in our mouths, on our skin, or up our nose to relieve pain.

The good news is we have so many ways to treat back pain.

The bad news is we have so many ways to treat back pain.

Most back pain is considered nonspecific low back pain, or NSLBP. In other words, we don't know why you have it. This is a potentially dangerous situation. If you are suffering with pain that limits your ability to function and makes your life miserable, you will be more accepting of any explanation for your pain and any treatment that promises relief. A confusing fact is that some patients will report pain relief with any pill, even ones that have no active ingredient. Studies have shown that most back pain patients are prescribed some medication. In one study, more than a third of patients were prescribed two or more drugs. It may be that by prescribing multiple medications, your doctor is covering more than one potential cause of your pain. But each drug can have one or more side effects, and all of them together may change the way you feel, while not significantly reducing your pain. Ideally, in most situations, one drug should be added at a time to see how it works before adding others. Since drugs are a standard part of care, we should understand how they are evaluated.

CLINICAL TRIALS AND PLACEBOS

By federal law, commercially available medicinal treatments for back pain (generally pills, but also liquids, topical preparations used by applying them to the skin, and substances that are inhaled) have gone through some form of testing to determine if they do what they claim. I can do a simple test by giving a back pain patient like you, desperate to get better, a pill that I say with assurance will help the pain. When I ask you to rate your pain after you've taken the pill, chances are you will report improvement no matter what is actually in the pill! There may be a real effect that reduces the pain. But your desire to get better, plus my assurance that the pill works and your trust in me, all contribute to your experience of relief. These factors unrelated to the physical effect of the drug are called the placebo effect. (The word "placebo" is from the Latin *plac,* meaning "to please"; the pill is pleasing.) Feeling worse in some way from the inactive pill is called a *noc*ebo effect (from the Latin *nocer,* meaning "to harm"; the pill is harming).

To control for this potential bias, attempts are made to minimize the effects of patient expectation and the relationship to the doctor. Comparison studies are done with the active drug, and another active substance, or with an inactive substance. In a good study, both the doctor and you don't even know which pill you are getting. This is called a double-blinded study. The goal is to show that the test drug is better than a known active drug, or an inactive (placebo) pill. This is important. Otherwise we would have Dr. Brown's Snake Oil, Magic Plantain Chips, and Desiccated Horse Manure, all demonstrating effectiveness in uncontrolled studies, and competing on the store shelf with acetaminophen and ibuprofen. You, the consumer, would have no way of knowing beforehand if one was any better than another.

As you can imagine, with so many variables that can affect how we respond to drugs, studies may have very different outcomes. If the majority of the published studies determine that the drug works, what can you expect in terms of pain relief from the medication you are taking? In other words, what is the definition of "it works"? If a researcher thoroughly reviews a number of similar high-quality studies, it is called a systematic review. Most respected guidelines for most treatments rely on these reviews.

The measures of success in one recent systematic review of drugs for back pain were 5 percent to 10 percent improvement, meaning small or slight; 10 percent to 20 percent, meaning moderate improvement; and more than 20 percent, meaning large or substantial improvement.

When you are in agony, a 20 percent improvement may be a welcome relief. But if you are anticipating a lot of pain relief with a drug that is suggested as very effective, you may be disappointed. Because of the frequent small changes with any one drug, multiple drugs may be given at the same time in the hope that the combined effects will provide more relief. I have evaluated many patients who were taking three or more drugs for their pain without good pain relief, but experiencing difficulties thinking and staying awake. As I have said, most medications will have some unwanted side effects. Therefore, more drugs usually mean more side effects. If you have had pain for years, you may have accumulated a number of drugs and their side effects, prescribed by more than one doctor.

Some of my patients felt much better just by slowly stopping most of their medications. I emphasize *slowly* because abruptly stopping a medication may cause withdrawal reactions. Speak to your doctor about the possibility of reassessing the medications you are taking, to see if some could be stopped.

If you have other medical conditions aside from back pain that require medication, the interactions of the various drugs could change their individual effect. This means that the addition of one drug to the drugs you already take could make you overdosed or underdosed. Make sure that your doctor knows and reviews with you all the meds you are taking and their interactions with one another.

MOST COMMONLY USED MEDICINES: EFFECTIVENESS AND CONCERNS

ACETAMINOPHEN (APAP), sold under the brand name Tylenol, can decrease mild to moderate pain. Its mechanism of action is not understood. It is frequently combined with another pain drug that has a different mechanism of action. Examples of this are with: oxycodone (Percocet); butalbital (Fioricet); and tramadol (Ultracet). The maximum suggested dose is 3 grams a day. That means about nine regular-strength (325-milligram) tablets or six extra-strength (500-milligram) tablets. Prolonged or excessive dosing could result in liver and/or kidney damage.

NON-STEROIDAL ANTI-INFLAMMATORY DRUGS (NSAIDs) are somewhat more effective than APAP. They are what they say: drugs to inhibit inflammation that are not corticosteroids. Inflammation is the body's response to *any* sort of injury. Steroid drugs, such as cortisone and prednisone, are strong anti-inflammatory medications, but they have more serious side effects than NSAIDs, especially if taken for a long time. NSAIDs—aspirin is one—inhibit the redness, swelling, heat (localized at the injury site or total body fever), and pain that occur with inflammation. Acetaminophen is not a true NSAID, because it only inhibits pain and fever. The two major side effects with NSAIDs are an increased tendency to bleed, because they interfere with blood platelets, which are responsible for clotting; and stomach irritation, because NSAIDS decrease the ability of the lining in the stomach to protect you from the effects of stomach acid, which could result in stomach ulcers. They also can make asthma worse, if you have kidney problems, can cause them to stop functioning, and can increase the chance of heart disease and stroke, especially if you already have heart disease or risk factors for it, such as high blood pressure, or if you take NSAIDs for extended periods.

ANTIDEPRESSANTS Some antidepressants are effective for many types of pain. They are thought to inhibit pain by increasing the available amounts of serotonin *and* norepinephrine, which are also important in combating depression. The antidepressants that only affect serotonin, such as paroxetine [Paxil, a serotonin specific reuptake inhibitor (SSRI)] and trazadone are not effective. Drugs that block the deactivation of serotonin and norepinephrine are effective because they make more of both available to the nerves. Examples are the older *tricyclic antidepressants* such as amitriptyline, as well as the newer serotonin-norepinephrine reuptake inhibitors (SNRIs), such as duloxetine (Cymbalta), which have a similar effect.

BENZODIAZEPINES [most often diazepam (Valium)] are effective for back pain related to muscle spasm. They can cause sedation and therefore some are used as sleeping pills. They can also be habit forming.

ANTIEPILEPTIC drugs may be useful. The concept is that overactive nerves in the brain and spinal cord can cause seizures, and drugs that can decrease this hyperactivity could also decrease overactive nerves that are causing nerve-type pain. Examples are gabapentin (Neurontin), topiramate (Topamax), pregabalin (Lyrica), oxcarbazepine (Trileptal), tiagabine (Gabitril), and lamotrigine (Lamictal). All have side effects, which may include dizziness, drowsiness, and weight gain.

STRIATED (SKELETAL) MUSCLE RELAXANTS may be effective for muscle pain. There are different classes of drugs that relax muscle. Examples that have been studied are tizanidine (Zanaflex), cyclobenzaprine (Flexeril), metaxatone (Skelaxin), dantrolene (Dantrium), and baclofen (Lioresal).

OPIOIDS block the release of Substance P (Chapter 3) and stimulate the release of serotonin. They include naturally occurring strong painkillers such as morphine (which are referred to as opiates and are derived from the opium poppy) as well as synthetic drugs such as meperidine (Demerol) and oxycodone (Oxycontin, Roxicodone). The opioids vary in their ability to reduce pain. For instance, codeine is much weaker than hydromorphone (Dilaudid) and oxycodone. All produce sedation, respiratory depression, and constipation. Opioids may result in serious dependency.

TRAMADOL (ULTRAM) AND TAPENTADOL (NUCYNTA) works on multiple systems. Tramadol acts like one of the weak opioids, in addition to promoting the release of serotonin and inhibiting the reuptake of norepinephrine (NE). Tapentadol is a stronger opioid-like drug and also inhibits the reuptake of NE. Although it does not increase the release of serotonin, when used with a drug that does, it can lead to dangerous levels of serotonin in the blood and cause *serotonin syndrome* (symptoms may include restlessness, diarrhea, increased pulse and body temperature, confusion, and poor coordination).

CORTICOSTEROIDS such as prednisone (Deltasone) have not been shown to be effective orally or by intramuscular injection.

In clinical studies, the drugs that appear to be most effective are NSAIDs and muscle relaxants for short-term use for low back pain, and tricyclic antidepressants and probably SNRIs for persistent low back pain.

VITAMINS, SUPPLEMENTS, HERBS

When it comes to herbs, vitamins, and supplements, there are fewer studies on which to base conclusions about their effectiveness for the treatment of nonspecific low back pain (NSLBP). Published reviews in 2008 and 2010 revealed that most of the literature on vitamins and supplements for NSLBP was lacking in rigor. Nevertheless, the use of the herbs devil's claw (*Harpagophytum procumbens*) and *Salix daphnoides, Salix purpurea, Salix alba*, and vitamin B_{12} injections all showed moderate evidence of effectiveness in decreasing pain. The herbs *Capsicum frutescens* and lavender oil had less convincing evidence of effectiveness. The National Institute for Health and Clinical Excellence (NICE) in the United Kingdom found, as of August 2010, that no vitamins or supplements have proved or been disproved to be effective for back pain. Just because herbs are naturally occurring does not mean that they cannot be harmful. There are many possible negative effects, especially if you are also taking prescribed medications. Vitamin B_{12}, however, appears to have no obvious downside. Glucosamine and chondroitin sulfate (GC/CS), previously thought to be helpful for arthritis, appear not to have a significant pain-relieving effect.

Supplements and herbs do not fall under FDA regulations, and unlike typical drugs, are not subject to rigorous controlled trials. A good resource to get scientific opinions about alternative approaches is the National Center for Complementary and Alternative Medicine (NCCAM). For more information, go to their website, http://nccam.nih.gov.

To further complicate the issue of medication is the fact that you may not be an average person. Published studies show the average effect of the drug on pain relief in a large number of patients. Some of those patients have little or no relief. That might be you. If you have been on a number of drugs or supplements for a long time, you may not be able to accurately determine whether you are getting any positive effect, and you might be getting only harmful side effects. Be thoughtful when taking medications. If you are experiencing improved function, without serious side effects or potential damaging drug interactions, then medication and supplements may help you recover to the point, let's hope, that you don't need them anymore.

ALCOHOL AND SMOKING

Alcohol and tobacco smoke, which contains nicotine and other potent chemicals, are two common substances not generally considered drugs. Living with back pain, you may have used one or both for relief.

Alcohol is a pain-relieving drug. It was one of the two drugs used during surgery—the other was opium—before the discovery in the 1840s of inhalable anesthetic agents such as nitrous oxide, chloroform, and ether. A stiff drink may reduce your back pain. However, if you are starting your day with vodka in your orange juice, you are in trouble. Alcohol abuse may damage every organ of your body, adding unintended problems such as liver disease, cancer, dementia, and hypertension. If you drink every day to decrease your back pain, discuss this with your doctor or a knowledgeable professional.

Smoking has no redeeming value. Even if you feel it calms you, studies have shown that smoking increases the risk of low back pain and of developing degenerative changes in the spine. Chemicals in tobacco smoke may reduce the blood supply to all the structures in your back, making it easier to sustain damage and harder to heal the injuries. If you have back pain and you smoke, you decrease the effectiveness of any pain treatment you receive.

CHAPTER 17

Choosing and Working
with Your Doctor

Most of you reading this book will conquer your back pain. Before it's gone, and for those with physical problems that will cause the pain to persist, it will be important to have a good working relationship with your physicians. Problems with back pain should first be discussed with a family doctor. He (or she) will have knowledge about you accumulated over time, which can be compared with your newest complaints and any evaluations that are indicated. He (or she) will be best equipped to screen for red flags. Since family physicians see so many patients with back pain who get better with little or no treatment, they tend to have a valuable conservative perspective. Your doctor may decide to refer you to a specialist if you have symptoms (your description of your pain and associated problems such as swelling and redness) and/or signs (physical examination findings) that suggest some special approach is necessary. Typical referrals from your family doctor or internist are to a physiatrist (a doctor specializing in physical rehabilitation), physical therapist, neurologist, *rheumatologist* (a doctor specializing in arthritis-type problems), orthopedic surgeon, or neurosurgeon.

You should be comfortable with any doctor or therapist you see for evaluation, advice, and/or treatment. We all have choices when it comes to medical care, even if they are limited by your insurance plan. Here are some things to think about.

A GOOD LISTENER

Chances are, you have nonspecific low back pain. It is important that you work with an open-minded physician who recognizes that doing the *least* testing and treatment may be the best course of action.

These days, doctors seem to have less time to spend with patients. Even though your time may be limited, it is important that you feel it is quality time. It is important that you are able to share your observations and concerns about your pain so that you provide a clear, complete history of your problem. If you're interrupted quickly, it may reflect a difficulty on the part of your doctor to listen attentively. Does your doctor look you in the eye as you speak, or is he or she answering the phone or looking at emails?

When it comes to finding help for your pain, your doctor's undivided attention is crucial. You haven't received the help you need because your pain isn't easy to understand. Physicians tend to diagnose based on their specialty. A good doctor will be able to say, "This story doesn't cleanly fit into my usual diagnoses. I need to look outside the box to help you." This is important in all of medicine but particularly in Pain Medicine. Too many patients are diagnosed as having a chronic pain syndrome without any real understanding of the reason for the pain. Your doctor's careful listening to your story may help uncover the proper diagnosis, based on your experience, not on his or her specialty. A very important study on back pain was done in 1984 by the Quebec Workmen's Compensation Board. It found that the treatment for the same symptoms of back pain with or without associated pain in the leg was determined by the specialist evaluating the patient and not by the symptoms themselves. The specialty of the doctor you see will influence the diagnosis and treatment of your back pain. A different specialist tends to do different tests and offer different treatments. Sometimes the best treatment is no treatment.

CLINICIAN OR TECHNICIAN?

We see a new doctor to get a fresh assessment. Just because you have a diagnosis that has been made by others doesn't mean it's correct. The reason you're seeing another doctor is because you still hurt. Sanford's pain (as you will read in Chapter 19) was diagnosed as first coming from spinal stenosis and after his failed surgery from the unique diagnosis, failed back surgery syndrome. Sanford was saved from a spinal cord stimulator or a morphine pump because he had an excellent internist who was open to a new approach and wasn't limited by the prior diagnoses. If you're referred for a surgery, nerve block, or spinal cord stimulation, a competent clinician will do an assessment before going ahead with the intervention. The person doing the intervention will be best able to determine when that intervention is not the best course of action. You want a thoughtful opinion before you proceed.

HUMILITY

Doctors are human. Humans are imperfect. No matter how great the doctor, everyone makes mistakes. There is no situation where anyone can be 100 percent sure of the diagnosis or treatment outcome. There is always an upside and a downside to everything that we do in medicine. You want to work with someone who is secure enough to admit to imperfection. It wasn't until I had been practicing medicine for many years that I could admit that I wasn't sure about the best way to treat a patient. I needed to think that I was always right. If another doctor didn't think that way, he was wrong. Experience has brought me humility. There may be more than one way to ease or eliminate pain. One obvious sign of a lack of humility is the new consultant speaking negatively about your former doctors. If the know-it-all doctor's evaluation and treatment are unsuccessful, he will have difficulty admitting it and working with you to come up with a new approach. My humble colleagues appear to be more friendly and kind—valuable traits that you will appreciate in your new doctor.

A thirty-five-year-old patient with years of back pain, whom I shall call Monica, had unsuccessfully tried three epidural steroid injections, the standard course for patients with back and leg pain. She was being managed by her orthopedic surgeon, who told her that the only option was to operate on her back to finally fix the underlying problem found on her MRI. Monica told him that she wanted to see if muscles might be contributing to the pain. The surgeon angrily told her that she didn't know what she was talking about. He saw one hundred patients a week with back pain, and if she doubted him, she should find another doctor. She did. After finding and treating the muscles causing her pain (not her spine or discs) she has been pain free for three years and is long-distance running again.

COMPLETE TRANSPARENCY

You have the right to know, before any test or procedure, what the downside risk is. There are no stupid questions. You rely on your doctor to provide you with the information that allows you to decide whether or not you wish to proceed with the suggested course of action. The details of the consent form that you sign prior to a procedure should be understandable. These forms are written by lawyers and are created in part to protect against legal liability. This is understandable in an environment where there are too many unwarranted lawsuits. But there *are* actual risks associated with most suggested treatments. It's not unreasonable to know beforehand what the intended procedure will do to restore your ability to do things that your back pain prevents and what is the anticipated duration of rehabilitation.

HELPING THE DOCTOR HELP YOU

If you're seeing the same doctor or therapist over time, make sure to talk about any changes in quality, intensity, or distribution of your pain. If there is a new cause of the pain, which is possible, you and your doctor do not want to be lured into believing that you're just treating the same old problem.

Sometimes bringing a friend or family member to the consultation will help you and your doctor. Observations from someone close to you may provide information that will help the doctor understand the impact of your pain and help you to recall the suggestions of the consultant.

The questionnaire that follows can be used as a guide to help you organize your pain complaints so that your doctor has a clear picture of what you experience. Your answers will suggest if more than a physical examination, such as imaging studies and blood tests, is indicated.

PAIN CHECKLIST

Define your pain.

Where is the pain?

- ☐ Neck/shoulder
  - ☐ Radiates to head
  - ☐ Radiates to arm
  - ☐ And hand
  - ☐ And fingers
- ☐ Low back
  - ☐ Radiates to buttock and thigh
  - ☐ Radiates to calf, ankle, foot, toes

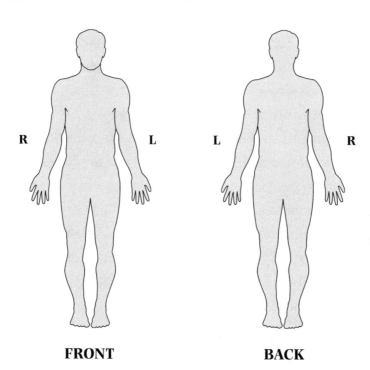

FRONT   BACK

My pain is:

☐ Constant ☐ Intermittent

Quality (circle):

Aching   Throbbing   Burning   Shooting

Stabbing   Squeezing   Stiff

Made worse by (circle):

Sitting   Walking   Lifting   Carrying

Standing in one spot   Bending over   Reaching   Lying down

Made better with: _____

Associated Problems:

☐ Weakness

    ☐ Where? _____

    ☐ What can't you do? _____

    ☐ Constant or intermittent? _____

☐ Falling

☐ Dropping things

☐ Loss of sensation

    ☐ Where? _____

    ☐ Constant or intermittent? _____

☐ Problems urinating

☐ Sleep interference

X-RAYS, MRIS, AND CT SCANS

Thoughtful back pain treatment should incorporate examining and treating muscles, the number one cause of back pain. In finding help, you will or already have discovered that many physicians do not think of muscles as the cause of your back pain. International, national, and local pain societies frequently ignore muscle pain in their publications and at their annual meetings.

Are you asked to get an MRI before the consultation? Overreliance on tests may make it difficult to find the real source of your back pain. Many of my patients have told me that very little time was spent on the physical examination before they saw me. Sometimes they were not even asked to undress. Despite indicating where they had pain and without a specific examination of the muscles in the painful area, they were told that the back pain was actually coming from another place, usually the spine.

You want to see someone who examines you where you hurt. Tests should be suggested only after having taken a thorough history of your pain and performing a physical examination, which includes testing muscle tenderness, strength, and flexibility.

PSYCHOLOGICAL/PSYCHIATRIC CONTRIBUTIONS

Living with persistent pain may result in new or exacerbated anxiety and depression. Getting appropriate help doesn't mean that the pain is "in your head" and is not real. Suggestions for a psychiatric or psychological consultation should be considered as a possible way to help you manage persistent pain. It is not an insult. On the other hand, we all have periods where we feel nervous or down. It's part of being human. I have seen many back pain patients on a variety of psychiatric medications for their anxiety and depression. After their pain was found to be caused by muscle and successfully treated, the anxiety and depression disappeared along with the need for the psychiatric medications.

CHAPTER 18

Dos and Don'ts of Daily Living: Sex, Food, Work, and Play

Tell them what you're gonna tell them.
Tell them.
Tell them what you told them.

(TIMELESS WISDOM FOR LECTURERS)

Let's review the things I've suggested to keep you healthy and pain free. When you want to refresh your memory about your commitments for a better life, you can consult this chapter.

First of all, if you cannot physically do something, don't do it. If you are asked to help carry something, for example, don't be embarrassed to say no. You may feel compelled to help; but if you strain yourself, it may result in serious injury. Remember, you are not obliged to be Superman or Wonder Woman.

Never use your back to lift. Lift by using your legs. They have the most powerful muscles in your body. In general, do not twist your body to grab an object that you want to lift. Face the object, bend your knees with your back straight, holding the object close to you. While your back remains straight, straighten your legs and stand up. When we lift like this, we are not using our back muscles to lift or to twist to position our bodies for the lift—both situations that could cause strain and pain. If you can lift only 50 pounds, don't attempt to lift 80 pounds. You can tear or strain a muscle.

When lifting is a job requirement, special care should be taken before you return to work. If you need to lift a 150-pound object with a coworker, then you should be able to lift close to 150 pounds by yourself to prepare for the possibility that your coworker drops his half of the object.

When having to carry an unusually heavy bag, divide the load. Carry two bags, one in each arm, so as not to strain the low back, arm, shoulder, and neck.

Avoid prolonged positioning. Any position held for too long stresses the postural muscles of your body. The older a person gets, the more readily this happens. (It helps to explain why Grandpa takes so long to get up from a chair.) Change positions every twenty to thirty minutes, even if only briefly, so that your muscles have a chance to move and recover their strength and flexibility.

OVERUSE OR WRONG USE OF MUSCLES

Avoid repeated and/or prolonged use of a muscle. Both can lead to immediate or eventual injury. Remember, too, that a muscle will have diminished capacity to perform its usual function if there is not enough time for it to recover from fatigue. This can result in sprains or strains.

Repeated overuse of a muscle may produce *repetitive strain injury*, also known as RSI. Carpal tunnel syndrome is a common example of RSI, which occurs when a nerve in the underside of your wrist, the median nerve, gets squeezed in the tunnel through which it travels (the carpal tunnel). Narrowing of the tunnel or swelling of the tissue surrounding the nerve results in pain, numbness, tingling, weakness, and sometimes even muscle damage in the hand and fingers. Typing and/or using a computer mouse for long periods is widely associated with the condition, but RSI has long been common in sports. Athletes know it as tennis elbow, or golf elbow, or baseball shoulder.

Whatever activity you do, you want to do it in a relaxed and fluid way. Training helps make you capable of the activity, both physically and mentally.

ADDING TENSION TO MISUSE OF MUSCLES

We often see cases of low back pain that might as well be called RSIWDRS, for "repetitive strain injury weekend driving range syndrome."

Consider this scenario: a stressed man (or woman) of any age gets out of bed on a Saturday morning with stiff, tight muscles from lack of exercise. Under pressure from work or possibly from problems at home, he heads to the local driving range and buys a bucket of golf balls, all to relieve his tension—or so he thinks. He starts swinging away, trying to whack the balls into the next county. With each swing, he twists his body. He jerks his shoulders, twists his neck. Suddenly laid low with what feels like an axe in his back, in absolute agony he stiffly gets behind the wheel of his car and drives home, where he gingerly climbs into bed to nurse the pain of the weekend warrior. Sound familiar? It should. It happens all the time.

IGNORING PAINFUL FEELINGS
PRODUCES MUSCLE PAIN

Emotional tension produces predictable patterns of muscle contraction. Having a feeling that weighs on you day in and day out stresses muscles unconsciously and may cause increased stress and tension in already painful muscles. As I have pointed out, when patients with pain are stressed out, they commonly feel that their pain gets worse.

Have the courage to be open with yourself about *all* your thoughts and feelings. Honesty with yourself may not only help you solve problems that seem insurmountable but may also help you reduce or eliminate your pain.

Now let's go through the specific dos and don'ts of daily living, starting at night when you go to bed.

SLEEP

Make sure to sleep on a moderately firm mattress. A soft mattress may result in increased back pain when you wake up. If your mattress is too soft, it inhibits the natural tossing and turning in your sleep that helps keep your muscles limber.

SLEEP HYGIENE

Sleep hygiene consists of the rules that sleep researchers developed to promote healthy sleep. Eight hours of sleep are important for your well-being. Most people getting a good night's sleep versus those that don't will report greater feelings of well-being, a greater ability to concentrate, and adequate energy for the activities of the day. Interestingly, they will also report less pain. Experiments on volunteers who are deprived of two types of sleep, rapid eye movement (REM) and stage 4, or slow-wave sleep (SWS), report increased generalized muscle pain, headache, and back pain with interruption of SWS. If your difficulty sleeping is intermittent, then occasional use of one of the typical sleeping pills may be helpful. If the sleep problem is long standing and constant, then you should get the help of a specialist in sleep disorders, generally a psychiatrist or a neurologist. Although we sometimes say if one is good, two is better, higher doses of sleeping pills tend to interfere with the slow-wave sleep, which could contribute to increased back pain. Another interesting fact is that anticonvulsant drugs such as gabapentin (Neurontin) and pregabalin (Lyrica) appear to increase SWS, which could be one of the reasons they reduce pain.

There have been conflicting opinions about the long-term use of sleeping pills, which are collectively known as hypnotics. All the traditional sleeping pills are in the family of drugs called benzodiazepines. Temazepam (Restoril), and the more recently introduced sleeping pills such as zolpidem (Ambien) and zaleplon (Sonata), which also stimulate similar areas of the brain to promote sleep, also tend to decrease slow-wave sleep. There are no clear studies that tell us how long you can take any sleep medication without being concerned about the effects of decreased SWS. Valerian root, touted for many years as a natural sleep aid, appears not to interfere and perhaps improves SWS. Melatonin, a hormone produced by the pineal gland in your brain, is related to the sleep-wake cycle and has been used by patients to treat difficulty sleeping. However, a study by the United States Agency for Healthcare, Research, and Quality found that it was not effective in treating most sleep disorders.

A variety of other drugs, including antianxiety medications, antidepressants, and drugs for seizures, have been used to help sleep. It may be a case of trial and error before you find the right one.

Try to go to sleep and wake up at the same time each day, even on weekends. Don't exercise less than two hours from bedtime. Avoid stressful interactions before sleep—you'll have plenty of time and more energy to deal with the problem in the morning. If you routinely have a drink late at night, it may relax you and even decrease your pain, but it also tends to awaken you in the middle of the night. Try avoiding alcohol close to bedtime. If you relax at night with a cup of coffee, you're not helping matters. Caffeine in coffee and many soft drinks will stimulate you and interferes with sleep. Napping in the evening has been shown in many studies to interfere with falling asleep and experiencing a deep and restful sleep. Force yourself not to nap in the late afternoon or evening.

Spending a lot of time reading in bed or watching TV may be further adding to your troubles. Ideally, your bed should be only for sleep and sex, but if you routinely read or watch TV to help you fall off to sleep, make sure that you are sitting up for both. Holding up a book will strain the muscles in your neck and shoulders, so use a bed tray with an easel to support the book, and only touch the book when you turn the pages. If you're not sitting upright in bed while watching TV but instead are lying on a pillow, you are producing an isometric contraction that puts excessive strain on neck and shoulder muscles. The last thing you need is to add more pain to your back pain.

For many people, sleeping on their stomach is uncomfortable. Try sleeping on your back with a pillow under your knees, or on your side with your knees bent and a pillow between your knees.

WHAT ABOUT SEX?

Healthy sexual function is an integral part of a normal life. Unfortunately, sex is often one of the first things lost when a person has persistent back pain. A healthy sex life creates a greater sense of intimacy with your spouse or partner. Many books and articles have been written about sexual positions to use when you have back pain. I do not have a recommendation about any particular position that will provide comfort for you during sexual activity. You should experiment with your partner.

I encourage sexual activity. What's important is not to avoid it. Life is never perfect; it's all about compromise. If you are not yet free from back pain—or if you are one of the few readers whose pain will not be significantly reduced or eliminated—it does not mean that your sex life is over. Forgive yourself for not being who you used to be. Unless you love yourself as you are, it will not be possible to love your partner as you want to. Remember, the most common form of foreplay is talking, which is sometimes harder than physical intimacy but often a necessary prelude. Successfully handling pain involves learning to master the art of compromise instead of abandoning yourself to defeat.

STARTING THE DAY

When you wake up in the morning, be conscious of the first thing on your mind. You have control over what you think, and what you think determines what you feel. If you want to overcome the disruption in your life from your back pain, you should try to create a positive attitude. It will allow you to see what is good and positive in your life.

Greet the day with hope, no matter what problems you might envision. Each day is a new beginning, with new opportunities. As long as you are not trapped in the illusion that today will be a repeat of yesterday, the day belongs to you.

If you feel stiff when you get up, the sooner you move around, the better you will feel. A hot shower or bath may ease back pain.

It is not unusual to have a hard time getting up because of pain and stiffness after a night's sleep. I have taught many of my patients to do the seven level 1 exercises for the low back (in Chapter 10) before getting out of bed to get them loosened up and then, after moving around a bit, to do all twenty-one exercises.

Dress comfortably. High heels can cause women discomfort. On the other hand, flats, which can overstretch calf and thigh muscles, may also increase low back discomfort. It's best to wear a shoe with a low, comfortable heel.

Men should never stuff their wallet into the back pocket of their trousers. The pressure on the muscles in the buttock may cause irritation and stiffness and sometimes even cause compression of the main nerve (the sciatic nerve) going to the leg, causing pain not only in the buttock and low back but also down the leg (sciatica) to the foot.

DIET

If you are sedentary and never exercise, your metabolism will slow down to match your low activity level. Therefore, to maintain a healthy weight, you need to eat less. But if you are tense and under stress, you're likely to take refuge in "comfort" food. When you increase your activity level, your body will burn more calories, and you may eat more.

I have had many overweight patients with back pain say to me, "Dr. Marcus, I swear I hardly eat anything," only to discover that whatever they were eating added up to too many calories.

Assuming that there are no other reasons for you to be gaining weight, the bottom line is this: if you are overweight, you are consuming too many calories.

Your doctor should check thyroid function, which is generally part of a routine comprehensive physical examination. Low thyroid activity (hypothyroidism) causes the body to burn fewer calories than it should. If you have this problem, you will find it hard to lose or maintain a normal weight, despite carefully watching your diet. Low thyroid function may also contribute to muscle pain. After the problem is corrected with hormone supplements, you may find your muscle tenderness and pain diminished or gone.

ERGONOMICS

Ergonomics (the word comes from the Greek *ergon* for "work" and *nomo* for "laws") is the scientific discipline of designing job equipment and a work environment to fit the worker. Proper ergonomic design aims to prevent repetitive strain injuries.

Here are some tips to help you analyze what you do each day and eliminate conditions that are hurting you:

The office space around you should be conducive to proper body movement. Computer positioning is very important. The monitor should be straight ahead of you, at eye level or slightly below; definitely not above eye level. The keyboard should not be placed too high, or it can bring on upper back and neck pain by interfering with the activity of the muscles in your shoulders and neck. Henry Z. Steinway, the great-grandson of the founder of the piano manufacturer Steinway & Sons, taught Hans that a good pianist adjusts the height of the bench so that the hands reach down to the keys. Same with computers: proper ergonomics dictates that your elbow angle should be greater than 90 degrees, so that your hands reach down to the keyboard.

If you use a phone frequently, use a headset. Do not hold the phone to your ear or cradle it between your ear and shoulder.

If you have an L-shaped desk, do not push off on your office swivel chair to go between each section of the desk. Repeatedly pushing off could strain your low back and hip muscles and cause pain.

When carrying a heavy briefcase, divide the load in two (equally, if possible) and carry one briefcase in each hand. This will lessen the strain on your arm, shoulder, and neck muscles, and will minimize the strain on your low back. If you carry a shoulder bag, consider a two-strap backpack instead.

Muscles are a source of pleasure when we are strong and flexible. Proper exercise allows us to participate in sports with minimal injuries. The next section is about concepts of exercise.

EXERCISING

"Is It Gluttony or Sloth?" Article in British Medical Journal *(BMJ) in 1995 about the obesity epidemic in the UK.*

As I look up sweating and puffing approaching forty-five minutes on an elliptical trainer, I smile at my friend Jack, who smiles back and says, "It builds character." Back in the locker room, the routine joke among the guys is: the workout is so much better when it's over than when you're beginning.

If it's a chore, which it often is, why do it? The answer is that most people don't. I exercise because I want to remain healthy and active until I die. I want to be energetic and think clearly. I don't want to have pain in my back, neck, and shoulders. I want to look trim. I don't want to be fat. I want to be prepared on my boat for any emergency that could be physically challenging. I want to sleep soundly. Exercise does all of this for me. Without exercising three to four times a week, I feel tired. When I feel tired and then exercise, I am full of energy. If exercise is so great, why isn't everybody doing it?

Before we had all the toys that allow us to get things done with minimal physical effort, we used our bodies for work, transportation, and recreation. There was a time when physical education was a standard part of our early education. It is no longer important. It is a snowballing legacy. The less each generation is connected to physical activity and sports, the less the next generation will be. We learn by imitation. If our parents were athletic, there is a better chance we will be too. Using our bodies is no longer a part of our everyday lives in Western industrialized countries. This lack of activity is one of the key reasons that we are faced with worldwide obesity. The other is consuming too much high-calorie food. In some of the countries plagued with famine, obesity is a sign of prosperity, and you may see it side by side with malnourishment. Being transported and having all your tasks done by another is also part of the same territory in developing countries where prosperity predicts obesity. Conversely, in developed western countries obesity and lack of exercise are more prevalent in the lower socioeconomic groups.

Is it sloth or gluttony? It is both. If we are going to reverse the trend in obesity, which is associated with heart disease, high blood pressure, stroke, diabetes, and osteoarthritis, we will need to change the way we live so that exercise becomes a routine activity that we embrace as a way of life. If you are obese, you probably don't exercise. If you don't exercise, your muscles will not be strong and flexible, and you will not be able to consume as much food as you would if you were exercising.

So is exercise always a good thing? Not necessarily. Anything we do in life requires preparation to do it well. If you exercise, do it the right way. I have seen many athletes who could run for miles but had a hard time crossing one knee over the other. Strength and endurance without flexibility isn't what anyone wants or needs. On the other hand, flexibility without adequate strength is not enough. Chances are you've tried at one time to start a regular exercise routine and didn't continue. You're not alone. Without understanding how muscles will react when asked to do more, it's not easy to get over the hump of the initial period of new exercise, especially if you didn't grow up as an athlete. Studies showed that, when asked for maximum effort, even individuals who already exercised moderately well performed progressively worse every day for approximately five days. Only after approximately ten days did they show improved performance. When you first start, don't be surprised if you get worse before you get better.

If you are a hardcore couch potato, the exercises I outlined in Chapter 10 are where you should begin. If you're already someone who participates in athletic activities, such as jogging, running, playing tennis, or golf, let's look at some basic concepts. Because most of us are squeezed for time, when we're ready to exercise, we can't wait to get into our physical routine. I am going to feel so good to move my body, or I know how good I will feel when I am finished, that I want to dive right in. Before we start any athletic activity, our bodies are not tuned up for the effort. We need to *warm up* first.

Healthy muscles that are prepared for a challenge need to be relaxed and loose. A relaxed muscle is not contracted because of tension and stress. The first thing we need to do is to address the tension that we bring with us. Breathing deeply and consciously, letting go of the tightness in our muscles (something I showed you in our exercises), followed by movement through the range of comfort, ending with a gentle stretch, prepares us for the rest of the warm-up. You might sit on a bench, extend your legs straight out, and kick them a hundred times as though you were swimming. Similarly, if your activity involves your arms, swing them back and forth as you might warm up on a cold day. You'll know you're warming up when you break into a sweat. Don't forget to cool down properly after the activity is over. If you're jogging, for example, and you finished the distance or time you had chosen, continue to jog at a slower pace that you will continue to decrease for the next three minutes until you are walking normally. Then do your limbering and stretching routine again before calling it quits. Above all, use common sense. Do not strain or exert yourself. May I remind you again? Don't try to be Superman or Wonder Woman; just have fun.

CHAPTER 19

When Exercise Alone Is Not Enough: The New News About Trigger Points and Muscle Tendon Injections

Y ou have already read in detail about three of the four reasons for muscle pain: muscle tension, muscle deficiency (weakness and/or stiffness), and muscle spasm. Now, as promised, here is the fourth reason: painful muscles that contain trigger points—in other words, tender nodules that you may have noticed when you pressed on an area of discomfort.

TRIGGER POINTS (TrPs), OR MYOFASCIAL TRIGGER POINTS

TrPs are tender nodular spots in muscles that are frequently associated with a taut band of muscle fibers, and when pressed will frequently radiate pain to a distant site. Laboratory studies have found evidence of increased electrical activity in the region of TrPs, and recent studies have reported pain-producing chemicals in the TrPs as well. Many articles have been written on the evaluation and treatment of TrPs, but there is diminishing interest in their importance—and even some authors who think they have no meaning. This is based on the inconsistency of evaluation and treatment approaches, which generally produce only partial transient relief of pain following injections of TrPs. It does appear that TrPs are important sources of localized and diffuse (widespread) muscle pain, but the lack of agreement on how to describe, examine, and treat TrPs makes it impossible to evaluate the many studies in a systematic way. This has resulted in TrPs and muscles not being considered in published guidelines for common pain syndromes such as low back pain.

TrPs sometimes benefit from injection—emphasis on *sometimes*—because an understanding of the relevance of TrPs to muscle pain underwent a sea change, at least for some of us, thanks to Hans, who was asked to treat President Kennedy's back pain after his trigger point injections were no longer effective.

Like other doctors, Hans injected TrPs to eliminate muscle pain—until he realized that half his trigger point patients were returning for treatment because the loss of pain was only temporary. Instead of concentrating on the TrPs, he began to focus his injections where the muscles attach to the tendons—that is, at the ends of the muscles. Hans decided to do this after a new scientific study demonstrated that this was where the muscle was most likely to be injured when strained.

I learned from Hans that successful elimination of muscle pain required injections into the ends of the muscle. If you have had injections into muscles and trigger points with only partial and/or transient relief of pain, not injecting the muscle attachments may be the reason that the pain returned.

The term "trigger points" has been used since 1921 to describe tender areas in muscles that refer pain to other muscles. Janet Travell (and, later, David Simons) popularized its use when she published papers describing the treatment of TrPs with injection of a local anesthetic. She further popularized the term "myofascial pain syndrome" in the 1950s. Although myofascial pain syndrome (MPS) refers generically to pain from muscle and connective tissue, it is frequently used interchangeably with the term "myofascial trigger points," contributing to the distortion that all muscle pain is due to TrPs.

It wasn't until Dr. Travell treated President John F. Kennedy that trigger point evaluation and treatment began to be widely used in treating back pain. President Kennedy's back pain turned out to be a study in comparing Janet Travell's approach to that of Hans Kraus. Although Dr. Kraus had successfully treated the president, predominantly with exercise, it was still generally believed that Dr. Travell's use of trigger point injections led to his recovery. When Kennedy was unable to walk without pain for months, trigger point injections given by Dr. Travell were actually ineffective. The exercises from Dr. Kraus addressed JFK's weakness, stiffness, and tension, and resulted in pain reduction and restoration of function. Kennedy was planning to establish a national back pain institute so that his own experience of success and failure with various interventions could be studied. But following the assassination of President Kennedy, the failure to distinguish between the two different approaches to treat back pain would contribute to the lack of acceptance of muscles as a legitimate area of interest for clinicians who treat pain.

TrPs became the world community standard rather than a comprehensive muscle evaluation and treatment approach, thus laying the foundation for overemphasis of TrPs as the sole area of interest in clinical muscle pain. With the introduction of sophisticated imaging such as CT scans and MRIs, clinicians believed that the source of pain could be visualized, minimizing the importance of the physical examination and relegating it frequently to a mere ritual. Many patients tell me their doctor did not examine them in the area where they reported pain. In those cases when an exam was done, muscles were ignored.

Finding the muscle that actually is causing your pain can be tricky because the culprit muscle or muscles will frequently refer pain to an adjacent or remote muscle or muscles, and on occasion the most unexpected muscle or muscles can turn out to be the source of the pain.

Moreover, if you have a large number of painful muscles spread throughout your body, identifying the correct muscle or muscles can be additionally challenging for physicians who follow the standard practice of pressing on muscles with their hands to find where the pain originates.

A REVOLUTIONARY BREAKTHROUGH DISCOVERY

Several years ago, I had the good fortune to join with engineers in developing a detector for pain-causing muscles. The Muscle Pain Detection Device (MPDD) is a hand-held, battery-powered instrument that identifies the pain-generating muscle by electrically stimulating the one that is actually causing the pain. An example is an athletic postgraduate medical student I treated who'd had ten years of low back pain that had been resistant to muscle injections and nerve blocks. Her pain was related in part to a muscle deep within her thigh, the adductor magnus, which ordinarily would never be considered. Being able to find the source of pain changed her life.

Examination with the MPDD requires that the patient is lying down, completely at rest, while the device is run along the entire suspected muscle from end to end. The following responses determine if and why a muscle is the source of pain.

- The suspected muscle contracts, but there is no pain. This tells us that the suspected muscle is not the cause of the pain. The muscle may be tender to pressure, but it is tender because pain is referred from another muscle or from an irritated nerve.

- The suspected muscle contracts, and there is pain. This tells us that this muscle is possibly producing the pain. The question is, why is this muscle in pain when the MPDD makes it contract? If the pain goes away with continued stimulation, this means that the probable cause of the pain is stiffness, tension, or spasm. These are problems we can address with exercise, electrical stimulation protocols, massage, relaxation training, and, sometimes, medication. But there is no need to do injections.

- When we continue to stimulate the muscle and the pain does not go away, it tells us that this muscle is a source of pain and that it has changed in some fashion. We know this because a stimulated muscle that contracts while at rest should not be painful. But if sustained contraction produces continuous pain in a muscle at rest, this is convincing evidence that we have found a cause of the pain.

The MPDD protocol is unique. It causes the muscle to contract and makes the muscle react in the same way it does as when the person has pain in real life. Most people with muscle pain feel relatively comfortable at rest, but when they move, they feel pain. When you move, you have to move more than one muscle at a time. This is referred to as a functional muscle group. It is difficult if not impossible to know which muscle in the group is the actual source of the pain. The MPDD offers the advantage of being able to move one muscle at a time, precisely because the MPDD is doing the moving for you. If the stimulated muscle is painful and all the surrounding muscles are not, it is reasonable to assume that that muscle is causing the pain.

A randomized, controlled, blinded study conducted at the Center for the Study and Treatment of Pain at the NYU School of Medicine found that the MPDD was much more accurate than finger pressure to identify pain-causing muscles. The two techniques were used to identify the painful muscles. The muscles were injected in the tender areas with lidocaine. This is the typical injection given for trigger points. Some doctors inject steroids, Botox, or saline. Studies have shown that it doesn't matter what you use when you put a needle into the painful area; it is the action of the needle that ultimately reduces the pain. Using lidocaine makes sense because it reduces the pain of the injection. Patients were asked to report the change in their pain and the improvement in their mood and function. The results of the study showed that muscles identified by the MPDD had more complete and lasting relief than those identified by the finger-pressure technique.

With the pain-generating muscle now identified, we can begin to eliminate your pain. As noted earlier, the areas of the muscle that are most involved in your pain are at the ends that are attached to the tendons. In these pain-producing areas there is an accumulation of pain-producing chemicals and a swelling of the tissue that squeezes the tiny blood vessels that bring oxygen to the muscle.

Only one muscle is injected during a given injection treatment. The needle has to be long enough to reach the spots where the muscle and tendon attach to bone, which is determined by the size and depth of the identified muscle. The treatment consists of using the needle to disrupt the muscle tissue, especially at the origin and the insertion. The interjections are referred to as a *muscle tendon injections (MTIs)* because of the significant difference in location of the injections versus trigger point injections (TPIs). An entire muscle, and not just a "point or taut band," is injected.

Fortunately, I was recently shown during a visit to Walter Reed National Military Medical Center that if prior to the MTI, I give an injection of ketamine (a powerful pain-relieving medication) and Versed, the MTI is painless. The description of the procedure may be upsetting, but there is no pain. After the ketamine is injected, iodine is swabbed on the skin over the muscle to sterilize the area. Then lidocaine is injected into the skin to numb the area. Five minutes later, the needle is placed into the beginning, end, and the belly of the muscle, and more lidocaine is injected. The lidocaine is used only for comfort and not treatment. The treatment is the needle in the muscle, and because of the ketamine, it is painless.

The needle injures pain-producing fibers, which then can grow, and bring in new blood. This flush of new blood washes away the pain-producing chemicals that have accumulated in the muscle and have kept perpetuating the pain; it also brings in much-needed oxygen. I repeat that it is the needle itself, not the injected anesthetic, which makes the muscle better.

Most patients immediately experience a decrease in pain and an increase in flexibility, but we cannot judge the outcome until all the identified pain-causing muscles have been treated. After one muscle injection, I typically provide three days of physical therapy to restore the flexibility of the treated muscle. Part of that therapy involves doing the first seven of the twenty-one Kraus-Marcus exercises.

Our records show that the typical patient who requires this treatment has four or five muscles that need injection. The entire procedure takes about two weeks.

A forty-two-year old private secretary, whom I shall call Alicia, had a two-year history of neck, head, back, and lower extremity pain after a fall. She saw many doctors, all of whom insisted that her pain was the result of bulging and herniated discs. Because she had diffuse pain in eleven of eighteen potentially tender spots, and had difficulty sleeping and concentrating, she was also diagnosed with fibromyalgia syndrome (FMS). Some of the doctors suggested that she undergo cervical and lumbar spinal fusions to address the problems with her discs, which they felt were the source of much of her pain. If this sounds confusing, it is. Many of the diagnoses for persistent pain that are batted around in the medical community are only speculation. If you have something on an MRI—say, a flattened disc—we can call that degenerative disc disease and say it's the source of your pain. If in addition you have tenderness in your upper and lower back, and a few other areas, we can call this fibromyalgia and say that it is also a reason for your pain. We have pills for your pain coming from your disc, and we have different pills for the FMS pain. You may be like many patients I see who have a medicine cabinet full of medications for the speculative diagnoses. The problem is, there is no definitive way to explain the source of your pain. Let's take a closer look at FMS.

Physicians have been baffled for centuries, with a group of patients, mostly women, complaining of widespread muscle pain and tenderness, and lack of energy.

CHRONIC WIDESPREAD PAIN (CWP) AND FIBROMYALGIA SYNDROME (FMS)

A subset of patients with muscle pain has diffuse pain and tenderness. The cause of widespread pains has been debated. Is the pain coming from the tender muscle itself, or are the nerves too sensitive, so that what would be felt only as pressure in a normal person is experienced as pain in someone with FMS?

In 1977, two Canadian physicians, Hugh Smythe and Harvey Moldofsky, reintroduced the term "fibrositis" to describe patients with widespread pain. They later renamed this fibromyalgia syndrome, when they described a collection of symptoms that included persistent widespread pain in at least eleven of eighteen specific muscles, fatigue, and nonrestorative sleep. FMS was originally thought to be caused by the tender muscles, but research suggesting overly sensitive nerves as the cause has moved the entire field toward the concept that FMS is a problem rooted in the central nervous system, resulting in muscle pain being produced even with minimal amounts of pressure. Patients with irritable bowel syndrome (intermittent pain in the abdomen with diarrhea and/or constipation, made worse with stress, without any evidence of disease in their bowel), chronic headaches, and chronic fatigue syndrome (CFS) have similar complaints or frequently also have complaints that could be diagnosed as FMS. Recent studies in patients diagnosed with FMS have shown that injections to specific painful muscles in one region of the body can reduce or eliminate pain in distant regions.

Imagine if your doctor has not looked for muscles as a possible source of your pain because of his comfort with spine-related and FMS diagnoses. If you are in the camp that says the pain is in your brain and spinal cord and we can't cure it, you may end up on FMS medication for the rest of your life. If you are in the bad-disc camp, you may be presented with surgery. If the pain was coming from specific muscles, no one would ever know. After years of ongoing pain and failed surgery, the pain could spread because of inactivity and attempts to alter your posture to make yourself more comfortable. With more pain, your mood deteriorates, and perhaps you will be put on more medication to manage both. If this is your story, there are millions in the United States feeling alone like you.

When Alicia came to me for a consultation, I examined her with the MPDD and identified six pain-generating muscles in her lower body. After I'd treated them, she reported that nearly all of the upper and lower body pain had gone. No other muscle injections needed to be done.

Alicia's case is not uncommon. Patients with disc problems visible on MRI who have diffuse pain may be told that they also have FMS. And it is common for someone in her situation to be told that a spinal fusion is needed. But Alicia's pain was not coming from her spine and discs, it was coming from her muscles. By treating the muscles that were actually causing the pain, not just where she was feeling pain, all of the pain in her body diminished. This is another example of central sensitization. She did not have FMS; she had muscle pain that, when properly treated, vanished. I have seen many patients who have been diagnosed with FMS who are now pain free after I found and treated the muscles that caused their pain.

I want to share a story with you about another patient who went through a failed back surgery. The words that follow are not mine. They are S.T.'s, a Manhattan publicist. When he heard that I was writing this book, he sent me this account of his case and asked me to present it. Here it is:

For more than four years, from late 2000 through November 2004, I suffered from excruciating chronic pain in my lower back and in my legs and anterior thighs. The pain was often unremitting. Day and night. Standing or sitting. It defined my life—and to a great extent, my wife's life. I was debilitated physically and emotionally. I work out of my apartment. I would have been unable to function if I had to commute to an office.

Walking was difficult and painful. I had to use a cane. At times, walking a block was a challenge. Sitting was painful. At times, my legs went into horribly painful spasms. I frequently had to go into the bedroom and lie down.

On some nights, the pain was so intense that I considered checking myself into the hospital emergency room and asking to be "put to sleep." I would have welcomed just about anything to alleviate the pain.

I consulted leading New York orthopedic surgeons, neurosurgeons, and pain management specialists. I had X-rays, CT scans, MRIs, and discograms. I was given epidurals, trigger point and steroid injections, and nerve root blocks. I received physical therapy. I also took Neurontin, an anticonvulsant medication often used for nerve pain and other medications. I was put on pain medication, including OxyContin, Percocet, and methadone. But I could never take enough to alleviate the pain because I had to be alert for my work.

I was cautioned that if I didn't walk often enough, my leg muscles could atrophy. So, I forced myself to take, despite the pain, long walks on the East Side.

An MRI had shown severe spinal stenosis in my lumbar spine, and it was recommended that I have back surgery. In May 2002, a laminectomy to decompress my spine was done. A spinal fusion was done with instrumentation, and a bone graft was taken from my hip.

The fusion did eliminate most of my back pain. Although I had some relief for two months after the surgery, my leg pain returned, and I was unable to walk, stand, or do any activity without severe discomfort. Unfortunately, I was no better after the surgery.

I received more physical therapy and epidural steroids, without benefit. I was told that the metal plates and screws in my spine might be contributing to my persistent pain and that I required another operation to remove them and to do additional spinal fusion.

I underwent a second spinal fusion in November 2003, and although I had a very brief period of approximately 50 percent reduction in my leg pain, the pain subsequently returned to its previous unbearable level.

The year that followed was marked by increasing levels of pain. The medication wasn't working. My internist, who was in charge of my hospital care after both spinal surgeries and who thinks "out of the box," prescribed a series of biofeedback treatments with a psychologist (mind-body specialist), which failed to alleviate the pain.

In October 2004, with the pain at an all-time high and my life more restricted than ever, my pain management doctor told me that my only option was another surgery to implant either a spinal cord stimulator or a morphine pump. And I was also advised that there was no guarantee that either would work, and that there was no way to predict the degree of relief if it did.

My internist advised me to be cautious and told me that he would explore alternatives. He phoned me a couple of days later and told me that he thought Dr. Norman Marcus, whom he had recently met, could help me.

I made an appointment, and I went to his website. Marcus's CV was impressive.

Despite his many credentials, I wasn't very optimistic. After all, I consider myself a very competent medical consumer, and I had been treated by some of the best doctors in New York.

After examining me, Marcus determined that my pain was actually from muscles.

He injected two separate muscles on two separate days, with a three-day follow-up physical therapy protocol after each injection. The injections and physical therapy resulted in a greater than 90 percent reduction in my pain.

I have been almost totally pain free for more than four years. I have not had a pain pill since the procedure with Marcus. I do not need a cane. My wife, Roberta, and I have a full social life. Three years ago, we visited the Grand Canyon and Southeast Asia.

In effect, Dr. Marcus has given my life back to me.

After what I've been through, I realize that there are countless other people in agony who, like me, may have lost hope. I've been blessed with pain relief. And I know many others can be too.

S.T.'s story is not unusual. Failed back surgery syndrome (FBSS) is generally considered to be a lifelong condition with some hope of reduction, but never with a full elimination of pain, by spinal cord stimulation and/or lifelong delivery of strong pain medication, orally or by injection. It doesn't have to be. At the American Academy of Pain Medicine's annual meeting in 2008, I presented a series of patients with FBSS. They were also successfully treated by first finding the muscle or muscles that caused their pain and then giving them the specific treatment that would diminish and frequently eliminate the pain.

CHAPTER 20

Other Cases of Muscle Pain, from Head to Foot, with a Stop at the Groin

B y now you may be thinking that if muscles cause most back pain, what about the pain in your shoulders or your elbows? What about headaches? Well, a pesky unidentified muscle can cause pain from head to foot. Not realizing this may lead to unnecessary surgery or surgical failure, resulting in more rather than less pain.

This is an unwelcome situation for anyone, but a career stopper for athletes, dancers, and others whose calling depends on a fully functional body. Professional lives are sidelined or ended due to a supposed torn rotator cuff or tendonitis—thought to be the explanation for a persistent sore shoulder or sore elbow—or a pulled hamstring, or any number of injuries caused by pain-generating muscles that can often be treated with the athlete returning to full function without surgery.

Here is a sampling of case histories of patients whose wide variety of pain was generally not thought to be the result of muscle problems and certainly not thought to be conditions that could respond to muscle treatment. When pain exists for years, as in these patients, it is often necessary to address all the reasons for muscle pain: tension, deconditioning, spasm, and muscle pain amenable to injection.

NECK PAIN

Sometimes you have no idea of the damage you can do to yourself. This is demonstrated by the case of a very bright, fit, and athletic twenty-six-year-old engineer we will call Jamy. His saga began in 2007, while he was working at a large manufacturing firm. The company president picked Jamy to work on an aggressive expansion plan. Determined to succeed, he worked on the plan for as many as fourteen hours a day—hunched over, head down—five and sometimes six days a week, for six months. Nothing else counted. "I was obsessed," he said when I evaluated him two years later, in 2009.

When Jamy finished the plan in July 2007, his head, neck, and shoulders felt as though they were tied in knots, and for the first time in his life, he experienced tension headaches. They rarely let up. At times his temples throbbed with what he described as "zap-like pain." In September 2007, given that his headaches were new, his doctor referred him to a neurologist, who ordered a brain MRI. When it showed nothing unusual, the neurologist ordered an MRI of Jamy's cervical spine. It showed no abnormality either. Jamy was then referred to an osteopathic physician, who, in turn, suggested a chiropractor, who provided physical therapy treatments as well as aggressive manipulation of his neck and shoulder, coinciding with the onset of pain around the first thoracic vertebrae just below Jamy's neck.

However, new problems appeared: jaw pain diagnosed as temporomandibular joint dysfunction (TMD); heart palpitations; and, as Jamy described it, "redness on the bridge of my nose, and thick, intense feelings of blood rushing through my head with any type of physical gym activity." One particularly puzzling symptom was a dizziness that he described as being similar to seasickness. Before all this happened, Jamy said, "I was able to comfortably visit the gym on a regular basis. These new symptoms started suddenly."

In the months that followed, Jamy was so out of it and so busy seeing specialist after specialist that he was forced to quit his job and to end a romantic relationship. His saga continued without resolution:

I saw two rheumatologists, three different ear, nose, and throat (ENT) doctors, and a dentist. The rheumatologists ruled out lupus and Lyme disease, and according to the ENTs, my nose was clear as a bell despite my persistent sinus headache symptoms. I had another brain MRI because I wanted to be safe. Bouncing around to more specialists led me to a pain specialist, who gave me weekly trigger point injections that only numbed my head for a few hours. Dramamine didn't work. Skelaxin and other muscle relaxers only made for more dizziness. I was baffling all of my doctors. Because of my jaw pain, I was sent to yet another dentist.

By July 2009 I consulted again with my general doctor, who put me in touch with a neurologist specializing in migraines. He diagnosed cervicogenic headaches and dizziness. Neck stiffness and TMD were clearly associated with my bouts of disequilibrium and the "out of it" feeling that accompanied my tension headaches. To alleviate some of the pain in the short term, the doctor injected Botox to areas around my jaw and occipital muscles. After the Botox wore off, I still had the same complaints—and the neurologist had me see yet another physical therapist.

The neurologist wanted to put me on antidepressants because clearly I was

showing frustration, though I chose not to take any and sought another opin-
ion from another dentist [for the oral and head pain]. I also saw three more
physical therapists and another chiropractor. All said to relax, that the pain
was in my limbic system in my brain and that I shouldn't spend any more
money on doctors; that I should take it easy. One doctor told me to go to the
beach; another said that I should swim; another said to take dance classes; and
another said to "read the Onion," *a satirical magazine.*

Seeing the new dentist was a turning point. She referred me to an acupunc-
turist that I saw in January 2009 and who provided the most relief, though tem-
porary, with trigger point acupuncture. He too was baffled by how persistent
my trigger points were. Stress alone, he said, could not be enough to cause such
trigger points in my neck muscles. It was thought that I had a form of whiplash
syndrome that was in the chronic stage, though I have not been in a car accident.
I had another neck MRI in December 2009, with the same results as before.
Thousands of dollars and hours have been lost. Most doctors had been baffled,
saying that everything was basically a result of an overactive limbic system.
My acupuncturist believed otherwise—that my brachial plexus needed to be
checked to see if a rib was pressing on it. He wanted another EMG done. Basi-
cally, because I am young and appear fit, my doctors did not take my problem
as seriously as they ought to or would if I were old and appeared out of shape.

In 2009 a neurologist referred Jamy to me. I examined him with the MPDD and
found twelve painful muscles on both sides of his shoulders, neck, and head that
had been misused during his six months of concentrated work. During that
period of time, Jamy's muscles had undergone almost constant sustained contraction. Jamy's symptoms then worsened as he made the rounds of doctor after
doctor for nearly two years without any lasting relief.

Although many of the specialists he saw felt that muscles were involved and had diagnosed him as having trigger points, none of the specialists were speaking the same language. As I explained in Chapter 19, trigger point treatment is muddled by a lack of agreed-upon methods to diagnose and treat the trigger point that is the suspected source of pain. After I identified the specific muscles causing his pain and dizziness in my examination with the MPDD, I treated Jamy with injections and exercise over the course of two months. The treatment was successful, eliminating Jamy's neck pain completely. He was also able to recognize that his obsession with work and other areas of his life was a threat to his health, and he agreed to see a psychiatrist.

SHOULDER PAIN

A patient whom I shall call Donald was a pitcher on his college baseball team when, for no apparent reason, a sharp pain in his right arm began to bother him during his sophomore year. The team doctor was baffled, as X-rays and MRIs revealed nothing. Donald saw doctor after doctor and embarked on a series of treatments—heat, ice massage, exercise, and ultrasound—but the pain intensified to the point where he was unable to pitch at all in his junior year.

Midway through his senior year, his uncle, a colleague of mine, suggested that Donald see me. My examination with the MPDD detected that the painful muscle was the right infraspinatus. I performed injections into the muscle and the areas where it attaches to the shoulder blade and the humerus. This procedure was followed by three days of physical therapy to relax his muscles and restore his full range of motion.

Four days later, Donald's pain was eliminated. After another week of exercises, he again had normal range of motion and was able to pitch successfully in three games. "I felt like I had a brand new arm," Donald told me. "The only problem was that the season had ended, and it was my last year."

ROTATOR CUFF TEAR/SHOULDER PAIN

The medical literature shows that shoulder pain is inconsistently evaluated and treated. Routine examination and treatment of specific shoulder muscles causing pain and stiffness in patients who are being considered for surgery for rotator cuff repair and impingement syndrome could decrease unnecessary surgeries and long-term use of analgesics.

An MRI found a full-thickness, buttonhole tear of the supraspinatus tendon on a sixty-year-old attorney with a two-year history of severe right shoulder pain and markedly restricted range of motion. Scheduled for rotator cuff surgery repair, Michael (not his real name) came to me to discuss what pain medication he could take after surgery to help him with his anticipated painful postsurgical physical therapy.

My consultation with him included a physical examination, during which I found six painful muscles in his shoulder girdle. A ketamine-containing cream, which can block pain nerves in the skin and that I use experimentally over an identified painful muscle, temporarily eliminated much of his pain and allowed him to move his arm freely.

Intrigued by this improvement, which suggested that muscles were an important factor in his pain, Michael asked me to start treating the identified muscles. Beginning with the most painful muscle, the supraspinatus, I systematically injected all the pain-generating muscles I had found. This resulted in eliminating all his pain and, after he did his upper body exercises for two weeks, total restoration of his range of motion. The surgery was canceled, and no problems occurred in the two subsequent years that I followed him.

GROIN PAIN

Some cases are truly extraordinary. A twenty-eight-year-old married business owner, who I will call Frank, suffered from pain in his groin and testicle. He came to me for a second opinion after his doctors recommended removal of his left testicle. Frank first experienced the pain at age eighteen while playing soccer. Although he had no obvious injury, the pain in his groin came and went for five years. When it persisted, he underwent varicocele surgery (to treat a painfully dilated vein that drains the testes). The operation gave him no relief. Three years later, at age twenty-six, he had exploratory surgery of the left testicle for continuing persistent pain. This surgery resulted in the removal of his appendix epididymis, a vestigial part of the epididymis, the structure that collects sperm from the testes. He had brief relief from the pain, but it soon recurred.

Then one day, while sitting on the toilet, Frank suddenly felt a tight sensation in his left hip; it progressed over the next month to the left low back and thigh. He reported narrow stools and a hard lump in the left side of his rectum. His doctor referred him to a gastroenterologist, who performed a sigmoidoscopy (insertion of a tube in the rectum and lower colon to observe any visible abnormalities). Nothing was found, but Frank was now diagnosed with spastic colon. He took fiber-containing laxatives and antispasmodics, which were ineffective.

The next stop, an orthopedic surgeon who diagnosed *synovitis* (inflammation of the tissue surrounding a joint) of the left hip. He prescribed physical therapy; that too proved ineffective. A urologist ordered an MRI of Frank's lower spine, nerve conduction studies, and a CT scan of the abdomen and pelvis. No problems showed up. Finally, after Frank's unsuccessful treatment with a chiropractor, his doctors said the time had finally come to remove his left testicle.

His internist hoped, however, that I might help him reduce his pain and avoid the suggested surgery. Frank had pain every day. It was so bad that he found it difficult to walk. On physical examination, he flunked exercise 6 of the Kraus-Weber tests, the floor touch. Bending over, knees together, and legs straight, he could not get his fingers to within ten inches of the floor. So it was no surprise that, when he lay down to do straight leg raises, he complained of pain in his hamstrings and buttocks.

His neurological examination was normal, but the MPDD identified six painful muscles in his low back, buttocks, and groin. After I injected the muscles, Frank was able to do all twenty-one exercises; and after doing them for four more weeks, his testicular pain disappeared.

Frank did feel an occasional recurrence of testicular discomfort over the course of the following months, but he recognized that his discomfort was consistently worse when he wasn't doing the exercises regularly. At the end of a year, however, he had no testicular pain while walking several days each week. On the days when he felt pain, he rated the intensity as two to seven on a scale of one to ten. But he could obtain relief with ibuprofen.

FOOT PAIN/PLANTAR FASCIITIS

A fifty-year-old schoolteacher, whom I shall call Kelly, was referred to me because of pain in her right knee and the sole of her right foot, along with occasional radiation of the pain from her heel, up her leg, and into her right groin. She also reported stiffness in both hips. Kelly described the pain in her right foot as intermittent aching and occasionally sharp, and made worse by running. She had been diagnosed with plantar fasciitis (inflammation of the thick tissue under the skin on the sole of your foot) and was treated with orthotics (inserts placed in your shoe to allow you to walk normally), which reduced but didn't eliminate the pain.

Kelly underwent bunion surgery in her right foot, and the pain she was experiencing in the arch and heel improved significantly for two years. Kelly felt that she could once again exercise, play tennis, and run. But when she did, the pain in her foot returned. She then saw a podiatrist, who diagnosed a flare-up of her plantar fasciitis. She stopped running and playing tennis and continued to use orthotics, but she had no relief. Kelly saw a sports medicine specialist, who prescribed physical therapy exercises and injected her right heel with platelets taken from her blood, a procedure called regenerative therapy. It had no effect.

Even though she complained of pain in her feet and ankles, I proceeded, as I always do, to check the muscles in the low back, hips, and thighs, since tight muscles in those areas can squeeze nerves that travel into the feet and cause pain. My examination found that muscles in Kelly's hips and leg appeared to be the source of her pain. The first muscle I injected was in her buttock, the piriformis, through which the sciatic nerve travels. When it is tight, the muscle can squeeze this major nerve serving the leg. Next I injected the adductor muscle in her thigh, after which the pain on the bottom of her foot was eliminated. This left only her heel pain, which appeared to be coming from the muscles in her calf that flex her ankles and toes. When they were injected, all of her pain was eliminated.

Result? Twelve years of pain from plantar fasciitis gone.

The cause of plantar fasciitis remains unclear. Current treatment options, which include nonsteroidal anti-inflammatory drugs, heel pads, orthotics, physical therapy, corticosteroid injections, night splints, shock-wave therapy (sound waves are used to break up knotted tissue thought to be the source of pain), and regenerative therapy (sometimes called prolotheraphy, which are injections into painful tissue to stimulate growth of new cells in hopes of diminishing pain), have not consistently provided adequate pain relief.

Muscles are a cause of pain, and if they are included in our standard of care, everybody benefits. From all the stories of patients who suffered for long periods, you can see that so many inappropriate evaluations and treatments were tried to no avail by well-meaning doctors and other health care professionals because they had overlooked the actual cause of the pain: muscles. Future studies should be done to see how muscle treatment can help others diagnosed with plantar fasciitis.

On the surface, the role of muscles and pain is obvious: "I hurt somewhere in my body, so chances are that is where the pain originates." You banged your leg on a door frame, and you see a swollen muscle or stretched skin that is tender when you touch it—that's where the pain originates. The same is true in areas of your body where you are not aware of some obvious injury. But you were injured, nonetheless, through the mechanisms we have reviewed in earlier chapters. Painful conditions, even though not generally associated with muscles, may still have a muscle-pain component, as we saw in the case histories of the patients.

What complicates things is the failure of our educational system to stress the importance of muscle anatomy to doctors and therapists treating back pain and other pains. Unless muscles are a standard part of any physical examination of a patient in pain, the opportunity for pain elimination will frequently be lost. Without a thorough knowledge of muscle anatomy, it is impossible to identify which, if any, muscle is the source of the pain.

The following individual is an example of a special kind of patient that I see. In such patients, a detailed understanding of muscle anatomy can lead to pain elimination even if they are thought to be suffering from fibromyalgia syndrome with years of baffling total body pain. If you are one of those patients, you too may have been prescribed medication that you could conceivably take for a lifetime, resigned to never being able to have a physically active and demanding life. Successful pain treatment in such cases is dependent on the understanding and belief that muscles can cause widespread pain and that, if properly treated, the pain can be eliminated.

Judy (not her real name), a thirty-six-year-old married mother of a seven-year-old daughter and a thirteen-year-old son, came with her husband by car from Alabama to New York to see me. Since the birth of her second child, she had suffered from pain in her neck, shoulder, low back, buttock, and chest. She met the requirements for the diagnosis of fibromyalgia: eleven out of eighteen tender points, difficulty sleeping, fatigue, and problems concentrating. Forced to spend days at a time in bed, she was depressed, tearful, and guilt-ridden that she couldn't be the active mother that she'd dreamed she would be. She was on six pain-related medications that she took every day.

Judy's lower body pain started with the second pregnancy. She had never regained her abdominal strength after her first pregnancy, even though she went to the gym routinely, mostly to work on the treadmill and to do light upper body exercises with weights, unaware of the need to strengthen weak abdominals. Her upper body pain began at about the same time, but she had some upper body discomfort for many years.

As I got to know her better, she revealed to me that her posture had been poor since puberty, when as a self-conscious adolescent she collapsed her shoulders forward to hide her breasts. Judy talked to me about painful memories of growing up in a troubled family. She cried. She got angry. She was able to see that her thoughts and feelings about herself affected the way she held her body and this, in turn, was one of the causes of her pain.

During treatment, along with doing the exercises I provided, Judy began to feel more comfortable in her own skin. It is hard to believe that she had forty-four muscles identified as causing her pain, and harder still to believe that when they were injected over the course of two months, her pain was eliminated.

Judy's story is very important because it speaks to those of you who suffer from total body pain and are on medications for years. You too may have many pain-generating muscles and associated psychological factors, all leading to a complicated yet treatable pain problem. Judy was able to get better because she never gave up.

CHAPTER 21

Not the End, the Beginning

D oes it sound reasonable that we can decipher the human genome, go to the moon, grow new cartilage in a petri dish, create joint replacements, cure testicular cancer, successfully treat HIV/AIDS, and not have a clue as to the cause of most back pain? If the number one diagnosis for back pain is nonspecific low back pain, referring to sprains and strains of muscle and other soft tissue, how could there be no mention of the evaluation and treatment of muscles and other soft tissue in the Joint Guidelines from the American College of Physicians and American Pain Society for the treatment of low back pain?

I know why. There are no large-scale studies done at multiple centers that demonstrate consistent responses to any muscle protocol for back pain. A national effort to understand NSLBP should begin with studies on how muscle and other soft tissue cause pain and how best to treat it. The crisis in back pain demands that this be started immediately. There is no drug company or device maker that will fund this because there is no product (drug or device) to sell. Most of the research in the United States today is industry-based research, meaning that some profit must be generated to justify research. If the government doesn't support this effort, the taxpayers will continue to bear the burden of a medical care system that is eating away our national treasure—and with less than optimal medical results.

There are also no good, consistent studies of surgery for backs with regard to strict criteria for patient selection and choice of type of surgery. The same lack of evidence exists for spinal cord stimulation, epidural steroid injections, facet blocks, radiofrequency ablation procedures, sacroiliac injections, and the choice of pain medication. The studies that have been done will frequently be considered successful if the patient has a 30 percent to 50 percent reduction in pain, and even less for medications.

New procedures that do not use new devices do not have to be approved by any agency such as the US Food and Drug Administration (FDA). Faced with ongoing back pain, we want to believe that any new approach is worth trying if we can escape the horror of endless pain. The patients who are worse after surgery or other procedures wish they had never gone down that path. What is saddest is that common sense has not been able to interrupt the juggernaut of the modern pain movement. Each year, newer and more creative ways to block nerves and alter anatomy are embraced by those who have not attempted to understand how untreated soft tissue contributes to back pain.

The medical school curriculum ignores the role of muscle in pain. Muscle evaluation is not part of the core training in physical diagnosis. Anatomy has been reduced to a ten-week course, when it is given at all. Many medical schools teach gross anatomy with computers and plastic models; the student never sees a cadaver. It's a worldwide change. In the United Kingdom, surgeons are being trained who have never dissected a cadaver. Anatomy departments are being phased out. We can imagine that we don't need to know the anatomy because we can see it with our high-technology imaging. We can't. The results speak for themselves. For back pain, we are going down a path of increased cost and decreased treatment success. We have stood the field of pain medicine on its head.

Pain medicine was created as a special discipline because of physicians' failure to adequately deal with the patient in pain. Multidisciplinary pain centers, which studies show are effective, can no longer be kept open because there is no funding. Insurance companies refuse to pay. The awareness that all disciplines are important in understanding persistent pain has morphed into lip service. Although more physicians are entering pain medicine each year, many (trained or not) wish to employ the newest injection technique but are incapable of examining a patient for muscle pain, or can't even identify the muscle that they might be palpating.

Pain medicine sprang from a collective awareness that mind and body are not separate. The most effective treatment of chronic pain had to address the whole person. No longer is that the collective vision of pain medicine. We emphasize costly high-tech solutions to pain complaints rather than cost-effective commonsense interventions. Yes, we need the skills of gifted physicians who can perform complicated surgeries and nerve blocks, but they should not be on the front line treating patients who need something quite different. Too many patients with NSLBP are receiving expensive, needless interventions.

Lack of exercise must be addressed starting in grade school. Physical education must be once again part of the school curriculum. Rather than spend all the millions of dollars on elite athletes who are at reduced risk of being deconditioned and obese, much of that money should go to our high-risk children. We must address obesity as a factor in contributing to back pain and a host of diseases producing suffering, disability, and escalating costs that threaten the financial viability of our health care system.

Some old war movies used to end with the phrase "This is not the end, it is only the beginning." My vision in our battle with pain would include an in-depth study of muscles in the educational curricula of all professionals dealing with patients in pain. This could result in many patients whose diagnoses leave them with persistent pain, unable to participate in their lives and on life-long pain medication, would be relieved of their pain and restored to normal function.

No longer would we accept a bewildering diagnosis called nonspecific low back pain, for we would be able to find the specific muscle or muscles responsible for the pain and have specific protocols to eliminate the pain. The cost of care of every common pain problem would decrease.

No longer would we be compelled to use expensive MRI and CT scan imaging or undergo piercing nerve conduction studies to find the cause in the majority of pain patients; instead we would be examining and treating their muscles. Inasmuch as imaging and nerve conduction studies will frequently show abnormal findings that do not actually explain a patient's pain, they should be carried out only to confirm a diagnosis, not to make one.

By looking first at a possible muscular cause of pain, we would decrease the number of unnecessary: (a) spine surgeries and their associated failed surgery syndromes, (b) epidural steroids, and (c) nerve block procedures and instead provide exercises and other muscle-oriented treatments to millions of people best served by inexpensive, safe, and simple interventions.

Doctors and other health care providers would be able to examine muscles and make a diagnosis. Many of the routine pain problems such as low back, neck, and shoulder pain could be handled by primary care doctors because the cause of pain would not be a mystery. Back and upper body exercises could be taught by office staff. In making muscles part of their practice, primary care doctors would be paid an added, reasonable amount, which would provide a needed increase in their income—an amount that would be more than offset by the savings on costly but unnecessary tests, procedures, medications, and, in the worst cases of all, the extraordinary expense of long-term disability.

To be sure, there will always be a need for specialists in complicated cases. But now, armed with the knowledge and skills to assess muscles as a cause of pain, unnecessary invasive treatments can be avoided. More patients could have their pain eliminated. With the elimination of pain and restoration of normal function, patients who were unable to function could once again have productive, satisfying lives. Everyone wins.

It must be done, and it can start with you. If you know that better care could be provided than what is now available, you are a force for change. Indeed, patients with back pain have already broadcast the message: 40 percent of patients with back pain do not go to traditional doctors because they do not get the relief they seek from them. In a way, it's up to you: ask your doctor about the possibility that muscles are contributing to your pain. Find a doctor who is curious about muscle treatment and whether it can help you. Empower yourself. You now have what most people lack: the understanding that muscles are the cause of most pain and the knowledge that you can find relief with simple, rational, proven, cost-effective interventions. You don't have to accept chronic back pain. Let us imagine that sometime in the near future we will all be able to look back in comfort and amazement at a bygone era of back pain treatment.

Acknowledgments

I wish to thank all of my teachers who have shown me that the more I learned, the more I needed to learn: the late Hans Kraus, MD, who taught me that chronic pain needn't last forever; thanks to Professor Siegfried Mense, who taught me how muscles can generate long-lasting pain; Arthur Elkind, MD, who welcomed me at the Montefiore Hospital and Medical Center Headache Unit; the late Edith Kepes, MD, whose vision enabled us to create at Montefiore the first pain center in New York City; Allen Collins, MD, who gave me the opportunity to start and direct the inpatient New York Pain Treatment Program at Lenox Hill Hospital; Rosie Faunch, who asked me to establish the Princess Margaret Hospital Pain Treatment and Functional Restoration Centre in Windsor, England; and Tom Blanck, MD, and Bob Cancro, MD, who believe, as I do, that muscles are an overlooked cause of pain, and who welcomed my work at the New York University (NYU) Langone School of Medicine.

I thank all of my patients, those I have helped and those who I was unable to help, for allowing me to experience how much could be done to eliminate pain and suffering and how much more research is needed. I am grateful to J. J. Herman, Clover Youn, and Kristina Pivazyan for their editorial assistance; Aya Araki, my office manager and friend, who always goes beyond the call of duty; Lauren Zander, for reawakening my imagination; and Suzy, the love of my life, who has taught me the meaning of loyalty and the essence of "never give up."

Attila Ambrus, Matt Wimsatt, and Begoña Rodriguez at TheVisualMD.com created the beautiful anatomical illustrations, and I am forever grateful to them and Alexander Tsiaras, whose commitment to improving health is an example of the positive power of social media. Thank you to Tim Bradley, who brought the exercises to life with his drawings. Thank you Sarah Durand, my editor, who kept asking for more, and Atria Books for believing in me for a second time and for enabling the unraveling of the enigma of back pain.

Appendix:
Resources, Recommended Readings

Societies, Foundations, and Organizations That Deal with Pain

AMERICAN ACADEMY OF PAIN MEDICINE
4700 West Lake Avenue
Glenview, IL 60025
847-375-4731
www.painmed.org

AMERICAN COLLEGE OF OBSTETRICIANS AND GYNECOLOGISTS
PO Box 96920
Washington, DC 20090-6920
202-638-5577
www.acog.org

AMERICAN PAIN FOUNDATION
201 North Charles Street, Suite 710
Baltimore, MD 21201-4111
888-615-PAIN (7246)
www.painfoundation.org

AMERICAN PAIN SOCIETY
4700 West Lake Avenue
Glenview, IL 60025
847-375-4715
www.ampainsoc.org

ARTHRITIS FOUNDATION
PO Box 7669
Atlanta, GA 30357-0669
800-283-7800
www.arthritis.org

CANADIAN SOCIETY FOR EXERCISE PHYSIOLOGY
18 Louisa Street, Suite 370
Ottawa, Ontario, Canada K1R 6Y6
1-877-651-3755
www.csep.ca

CHRONIC PAIN OUTREACH ASSOCIATION
www.chronicpain.org

FIBROMYALGIA NETWORK
PO Box 31750
Tucson, AZ 85751-1750
800-853-2929
www.fmnetnews.com

THE COCHRANE LIBRARY
www.cochrane.org

THE VISUAL MD
www.thevisualmd.com

Articles That May Be of Interest

Ge, H-Y, Wang Y, Danneskiold-Samsøe, B, Graven-Nielsen, T, Arendt-Nielsen, L. "The Predetermined Sites of Examination for Tender Points in Fibromyalgia Syndrome are Frequently Associated with Myofascial Trigger Points." *Journal of Pain* 11, no. 7 (2010):644–51.

Ge, H-Y, Nie, H, Madeleine, P, Danneskiold-Samsøe, B, Graven-Nielsen, T, Arendt-Nielsen, L. "Contribution of the Local and Referred Pain from Active Myofascial Trigger Points in Fibromyalgia Syndrome." *Pain* 147, no. 1–3 (2009): 233–40.

Martin, BI, Deyo, RA, Mirza, SK, et al. "Expenditures and Health Status Among Adults with Back and Neck Problems." *JAMA* 299, no. 6 (2008):656–64.

Deyo, RA, Weinstein, JN. "Primary Care—Low Back Pain." *New England Journal of Medicine* 344, no. 5 (2001):363–70.

Carragee, EJ, Cohen, SP. "Lifetime Asymptomatic for Back Pain: The Validity of Self-Report Measures in Soldiers." *Spine* 34, no. 9 (2009): 978–83.

Marcus, NJ, Gracely, E, O'Keefe, K. "A Comprehensive Protocol to Diagnose and Treat Pain of Muscular Origin May Successfully and Reliably Decrease or Eliminate Pain in a Chronic Pain Population." *Pain Medicine* 11, no. 1 (2010): 25–34.

Recommended Books

FREEDOM FROM PAIN
Norman Marcus, MD, and Jean Arbeiter

> A comprehensive approach to manage pain that won't go away.

INTO THE UNKNOWN
Susan Schwartz

> This book discusses the life and studies of Dr. Hans Kraus, who was my teacher and mentor and the pioneer of sports medicine.

PRESIDENT KENNEDY: PROFILE IN POWER
Richard Reeves

> The details of President Kennedy's life, including the treatment of his back pain by Dr. Hans Kraus and Dr. Janet Travell, are elucidated in this book.

BACKACHE, STRESS, AND TENSION: THEIR CAUSE, PREVENTION, AND TREATMENT
Hans Kraus, MD

> Classic text on commonsense approaches to back pain.

THE MIND-BODY PRESCRIPTION
John Sarno, MD

> Dr. Sarno deals with the mind-body connection in back pain.

FUNDAMENTALS OF MUSCULOSKELETAL PAIN
Thomas Graven-Nielsen, Lars Arendt-Nielsen, and Siegfried Mense

> Published by IASP Press and edited by prominent muscle researchers, this is a scholarly synopsis of the muscular contributions to musculoskeletal pain.

THE STRUCTURE OF SCIENTIFIC REVOLUTIONS
Thomas S. Kuhn

> One of the most important books on the philosophy of change in science.
> Not for the fainthearted.

MUSCLE PAIN: UNDERSTANDING THE MECHANISMS
Siegfried Mense, MD, and Robert Gerwin

> If you're interested in dense neuroscience, this is for you.

ATLAS OF ANATOMY
Published by Thieme

> One of the best collections of anatomical drawings to help understand
> muscle anatomy.

*HOPE OR HYPE: THE OBSESSION WITH MEDICAL ADVANCES
AND THE HIGH COST OF FALSE PROMISES*
Richard Deyo, MD

> A critical look at the illusion of progress in medical care; important at this
> time of financial stress in health care.

TAKING THE MEDICINE
Druin Burch

> The history and importance of evidence-based medicine.

Stress/Pain Management Guided Imagery

CD and Tapes by Belleruth Naparstek
http://belleruthnaparstek.com

Bibliography

Buscemi, N., B. Vandermeer, R. Pandya, N. Hooton, T.L. Tjosvold, L. Hartling, G. Baker, S. Vohra, and T. Klassen. "Melatonin for Treatment of Sleep Disorders." Evidence Report/Technology. Assessment No. 108. Prepared by the University of Alberta Evidence-Based Practice Center, under Contract No. 290–02–0023, 2004.

Charifi, N., K. Fawzi, L. Feasson, and C. Denis. "Effects of Endurance Training on Satellite Cell Frequency in Skeletal Muscle of Old Men." *Muscle & Nerve* 28 (2003): 87–92.

Chou, R., and L. Hoyt Huffman. "Medications for Acute and Chronic Low Back Pain: A Review of the Evidence for an American Pain Society/American College of Physicians Clinical Practice Guideline." *Annals of Internal Medicine* 147, no. 7 (October 2, 2007): 505–14.

Chou, R., A. Qaseem, D.K. Owens, P. Shekelle, and for the Clinical Guidelines Committee of the American College of Physicians. "Diagnostic Imaging for Low Back Pain: Advice for High-Value Health Care from the American College of Physicians." *Annals of Internal Medicine* 154, no. 3 (February 1, 2011): 181-89.

Deyo, R.A., D.T. Gray, W. Kreuter, S. Mirza, and B.I. Martin. "United States Trends in Lumbar Fusion Surgery for Degenerative Conditions." *Spine* 30, no. 12 (2005): 1441–47.

Deyo, R.A., and J.N. Weinstein. "Low Back Pain." *The New England Journal of Medicine* 344, no. 5 (2001): 363–70.

Fine, P., K. Burgio, D. Borell-France, H. Richter, W. Whitehead, A. Weber, and M. Brown. "Teaching and Practicing of Pelvic Floor Muscle Exercises in Primiparous Women During Pregancy and Postpartum Period." *American Journal of Obstetrics and Gynecology* 197 (2007): 33.

Fussenegger, D., A. Pietrobelli, and K. Widhalm. "Childhood Obesity: Political Developments in Europe and Related Perspectives for Future Action on Prevention." *Obesity Reviews* 9, no. 1 (2008): 76–82.

Gagnier, J. J. "Evidence Based Review of Natural Health Products for Non-Specific Low Back Pain." *The Open Pain Journal* 3 (2010): 52–9.

Gagnier, J. J. "Evidence-Informed Management of Chronic Low Back Pain with Herbal, Vitamin, Mineral, and Homeopathic Supplements." *The Spine Journal* 8, no. 1 (2008): 70–79.

Gagnier, J. J., H. Boon, P. Rochon, D. Moher, J. Barnes, C. Bombardier, and for the CONSORT Group*. "Reporting Randomized, Controlled Trials of Herbal Interventions: An Elaborated Consort Statement." *Annals of Internal Medicine* 144, no. 5 (March 7, 2006): 364–67.

Gagnier, J. J., D. Moher, H. Boon, J. Beyene, and C. Bombardier. "Randomized Controlled Trials of Herbal Interventions Underreport Important Details of the Intervention." *Journal of Clinical Epidemiology* 64, no. 7 (2011): 760–69.

Gaston, A., and A. Cramp. "Exercise During Pregnancy: A Review of Patterns and Determinants." *Journal of Science and Medicine in Sport* 14, no. 4 (2011): 299–305.

Graven-Nielsen, T., L. Arendt-Nielsen, and S. Mense. "Fundamentals of Musculoskeletal Pain." 160–61. Seattle: IASP Press, 2008.

Hunter, C., M. Dubois, S. Zou, W. Oswald, K. Coakley, M. Shehebar, and A. M. Conlon. "A New Muscle Pain Detection Device to Diagnose Muscles as a Source of Back and/or Neck Pain." *Pain Med* 11, no. 1 (Jan 2010): 35–43.

IASP. *Core Curriculum*. 3rd ed. Seattle: IASP Press, 2005.

Kadi, F. N. Charifi, C. Denis, and J. Lexell. "Satellite Cells and Myonuclei in Young and Elderly Women and Men." *Muscle & Nerve* 29 (2004): 120–27.

Kadi, F., and E. Ponsot. "The Biology of Satellite Cells and Telomeres in Human Skeletal Muscle: Effects of Aging and Physical Activity." *Scandinavian Journal of Medicine and Science in Sports* 20 (2010): 39–48.

Kori, S. H., R. P. Miller, and D. D. Todd, "Kinisiophobia: A New View of Chronic Pain Behavior." *Pain Management*, Jan/Feb (1990): 35–43.

Kraus, H. *Backache, Stress, & Tension*. New York: Pocket Books, 1965.

Kraus, H. *Diagnosis and Treatment of Muscle Pain*. Chicago: Quintessence Books, 1988.

Kraus, H., W. Nagler, and A. Melleby. "Evaluation of an Exercise Program for Back Pain." *American Family Physician* 28, no. 3 (1983): 153–58.

Mackey, A. L., B. Esmarck, F. Kadi, S. O. Koskinen, M. Kongsgaard, A. Sylvestersen, J. J. Hansen, G. Larsen, and M. Kjaer. "Enhanced Satellite Cell Proliferation with Resistance Training in Elderly Men and Women." *Scand J Med Sci Sports* 17, no. 1 (Feb 2007): 34–42.

Marcus, N.J., E. Gracely, and K.O. Keefe. "A Comprehensive Protocol to Diagnose and Treat Pain of Muscular Origin May Successfully and Reliably Decrease or Eliminate Pain in a Chronic Pain Population." *Pain Medicine* 11, no. 1 (2010): 25–34.

Marcus, N.J., and S. Mense, "Muscle Pain." *Principles and Practice of Pain Medicine.* Ed. Z. H. Bajwa, J. Wootton, C. Warfield, McGraw-Hill. In Press.

Marcus, N.J., and J. Ough, "Evaluation and Treatment of Muscle Pain." *Pain Medicine.* Ed. Belval, B. Springer. In Press.

Martin, B.I., R.A. Deyo, S.K. Mirza, J.A. Turner, B.A. Comstock, W. Hollingworth, and S.D. Sullivan. "Expenditures and Health Status among Adults with Back and Neck Problems." *JAMA* 299, no. 6 (2008): 656–63.

Mayer, E.A., and M.C. Bushnell, eds. *Functional Pain Syndromes: Presentation and Pathophysiology.* Seattle: IASP Press, 2009.

Mense, S., and R.D. Gerwin. *Muscle Pain: Understanding the Mechanisms.* 1st ed. Heidelberg: Springer, 2010.

Mense, S., D.G. Simons, and I.J. Russell. *Muscle Pain: Understanding Its Nature, Diagnosis, and Treatment.* Philadelphia: Lippincott Williams & Wilkins, 2001.

Mørkved, S., K. Bø, B. Schei, and K.Å. Salvesen. "Pelvic Floor Muscle Training During Pregnancy to Prevent Urinary Incontinence: A Single-Blind Randomized Controlled Trial." *Obstetrics & Gynecology* 101, no. 2 (2003): 313–19.

Owe, K. M., W. Nystad, and K. Bø. "Correlates of Regular Exercise During Pregnancy: The Norwegian Mother and Child Cohort Study." *Scand J Med Sci Sports* 19, no. 5 (2009): 637–45.

Pearson, S.J., A. Young, A. Macaluso, G. Devito, M.A. Nimmo, M. Cobbold, and S.D.R. Harridge. "Muscle Function in Elite Weightlifters." *Applied Sciences: Physical Fitness and Performance* 34 (2002): 1199–206.

Sacks, F., G.A. Bray, V.J. Carey, S.R. Smith, D.H. Ryan, S.D. Anton, K. McManus, *et al.* "Comparison of Weight Loss Diets with Different Compositions of Fat

Protein and Carbohydrates." *The New England Journal of Medicine* 360, no. 9 (2009): 859–73.

Stuge, B., E. Laerun, G. Kirkesola, and N. Vollestad. "The Efficacy of a Treatment Program Focusing on Specific Stabilizing Exercises for Pelvic Girdle Pain after Pregnancy." *Spine* 29 (2004): 351–59.

van Middelkoop, M., S.M. Rubinstein, A.P. Verhagen, R.W. Ostelo, B.W. Koes, and M.W. van Tulder. "Exercise Therapy for Chronic Nonspecific Low-Back Pain." *Best Practice & Research Clinical Rheumatology* 24, no. 2 (2010): 193–204.

Verbunt, J.A., H.A. Seelen, J.W. Vlaeyen, E.J. Bousema, G.J. van der Heijden, P.H. Heuts, and J.A. Knottnerus. "Pain-Related Factors Contributing to Muscle Inhibition in Patients with Chronic Low Back Pain: An Experimental Investigation Based on Superimposed Electrical Stimulation." *Clinical Journal of Pain* 21, no. 3 (May–Jun 2005): 232–40.

Index